Coronavirus on My Mind

The Journey of an ER Doc into the Madness of COVID-19

Copyright © 2020 by Xavier Odili, MD
All rights reserved. No part of this book may be reproduced, scanned, or distributed in any printed or electronic form without permission.
First Edition: April 2020
Second Edition: June 2020
Published by The Book Patch, LLC – http://thebp.site/228081
Printed in the United States of America
ISBN: 978-16-4858-1601

Coronavirus on My Mind

The Journey of an ER Doc into the Madness of COVID-19

by
Dr. Xavier Odili

This book is dedicated to my wife, the hardest working woman I know. When I'm on a 24-hour shift over the weekend, she is the primary caregiver for our 4 boys. At home, there are no call rooms and no coffee breaks – she does the job often with little sleep. As hard as I work, I know she works even harder. I appreciate every sacrifice she makes for our family. Without her, nothing I do is possible. Thank you.

Dr. Xavier Odili

WARNING:

THE CONTENTS OF THIS BOOK ARE NOT MEANT FOR EVERYONE. READ AT YOUR OWN RISK.

Table of Contents

Introduction ix

Preparing the Mind for the Fight to Come 1

Something Wicked This Way Comes 3

Outbreak 8

Containing the Contagion 24

Leading the World 53

The USA Collectively Holds its Breath 94

As the Death Toll Rises 112

The Second Wave of COVID-19 Cometh 120

The Truth and Myths of Coronavirus 131

Dr. Xavier Odili

A Physician's Plea

We have known for months that the working class, the women of our country, and the peoples of color in America are at higher risk of contracting COVID-19 for many reasons. The types of jobs that cannot be performed from home, the types of jobs where social distancing is nearly impossible, and the home life situations where an infected person cannot distance from family to protect them all contribute to that increased risk. We also know that the differences in the way some people in these groups access and interact with our healthcare system that led to higher rate of death in minorities from diabetes and heart disease would translate into higher death rate from COVID-19 as well. Despite these facts, we are seeing a crisis of misinformation spreading faster than the virus. Some people don't believe the virus is real. Some people don't think the virus is hurting anyone. Some people think the death toll is exaggerated. The images of large crowds of people at parties and inside bars and clubs are disturbing. As a healthcare provider, I plead to you today to think twice before you underestimate this virus. If not for yourself, then for your neighbors, your extended family, and your coworkers. You may not die from a COVID-19 infection, in fact, you may not even notice if you are infected, but if you pass the infection to a friend or family member who isn't as lucky, you can't take that back. The truths of COVID-19 must be spread to dispel the rumors and myths in hopes that we continue to slow the spread of infection until a vaccine is developed.

Introduction

We are in the fight of our lifetime. I hesitated several times before deciding to put this out, because this is a crisis and people are living through it and because we don't know when this will end. The truth is raw and not everyone is ready to face it. The stories told in this book are real. Ultimately, I realized that organizing my thoughts and feelings helped me deal with the stress of dealing with an infection that was changing the whole world and the daily life of my family and friends, and that others might feel reassured to know that they are not alone in their fears. Although this started as a record of my thoughts, I realized that the daily conversations with patients, friends, and family were all about reinforcing the truth and rejecting false information about this epidemic.

I've only been practicing emergency medicine for about 10 years, so I've never seen anything like what we're facing. Swine Flu, SARS, MERS, Ebola ... none of these affected our country the way the novel Coronavirus is changing our lives. In this time of rapid change and uncertainty, telling the difference between fact and fiction is so difficult. Every day I spend hours educating family, friends, neighbors, and patients on the truth and dispelling myths in hopes that they will continue spreading truth to their family and friends.

After reading this book, you will probably learn a lot about COVID-19. This new virus has changed life for everyone so quickly, it can seem hard to keep up. There are lots of myths about the virus I plan to dispel and misconceptions I hope to clarify for you. It's amazing how fast misinformation spreads. Despite the fear and uncertainty, I still have hope that together, as a nation, we will find reassurance with facts instead of giving in to fear and work together to do everything necessary to overcome this pandemic.

Chapter 1

Preparing the Mind for the Fight to Come

It seems as if a different virus threatens the world every few years. Whether it's a novel mutation of a previously common disease like H1N1 Influenza, or a re-emergence of an old disease like Ebola, a new epidemic can cause significant concern around the globe. During the Ebola outbreak, I remember being worried about the virus reaching our country via an international traveler. I remember the rush for hospitals to acquire the appropriate protective equipment for staff. I remember the calls for everyone to be vigilant and look for patients with signs and symptoms of Ebola virus - bloody discharge from eyes, nose, mouth, bloody diarrhea, etc. Despite all this, a man who had recently returned from Liberia in western Africa presented to an ER in Dallas complaining of mild but similar symptoms and was evaluated, then sent home. His symptoms worsened and he went to another hospital and later the diagnosis was made.

Dozens of people were exposed while this patient was in our country and fears of an outbreak ran wild. Fortunately for us, the spread of the disease required physical contact with bodily fluids and the symptoms of Ebola manifest relatively quickly, so we never saw those isolated cases evolve into a pandemic. Because the symptoms are so different from our common seasonal illnesses, the other patients with Ebola were identified quickly and isolated from the general public. Although Ebola has been spreading in Central and West Africa for decades, after spreading into Europe in 2014 and halfway across the globe to the US, we soon saw the development of new anti-viral drugs and a possible vaccine. When people of the world work together, we can achieve great things.

Innovation, cooperation, and communication. These are the tools that the scientific and medical community use to combat the uncertainty of a new infection. Trust in the scientific method and faith in our local and national leadership will strengthen our resolve along the course of this new journey. Keeping in mind that the actions of individuals have long-lasting effects on everyone, we must endeavor to make choices for the greater good. Each step forward toward a brighter future is a step we must take together.

Chapter 2

Something Wicked This Way Comes

December 31, 2019

I was off on New Year's Eve for the first time in many years. I'm married with four children, so I really try to make the most of my time off and spend it with family. I was scheduled for a 24-hour shift on New Year's Day, so I stayed home with my wife and kids, ordered some food, watched some of the TV celebrations and watched the neighborhood fireworks from our driveway. Meanwhile, China was informing the world for the first time about a group of patients with pneumonia who all were all in close proximity of a seafood and meat market in Wuhan, Hubei Province of China. This was not the first time a new illness had appeared in a foreign land and it will probably not be the last, but I definitely was not paying attention to this reporting at the time.

In a perfect world, someone would have noticed this outbreak and advised the government to assess our country's preparedness for a pandemic. On this side of the Pacific, we were making resolutions for the new year, anticipating the most likely Super Bowl matchups, and thinking ahead to summer vacation plans. Ignorance truly is bliss.

January 20, 2020

News outlets are reporting that a patient near Seattle, Washington has tested positive for Coronavirus, the first patient to be confirmed by CDC lab testing. According to the case report published by the New England Journal of Medicine, the patient returned to the US from Wuhan, China on January 15 after a family visit. On January 19, he went to an urgent care clinic with a 4-day history of cough and fever. At the clinic, he had a fever, a rapid heart rate, and a mild elevation in blood pressure. He tested negative for the flu. Because of his travel history, the local health department was notified, swabs were collected for testing, and the patient was sent home to quarantine with monitoring by the local health department. On January 20, the CDC reported the swabs tested positive for COVID-19.

The public was never given information about where this person worked or how many people he came into contact with between January 15 and January 19. Like other outbreaks in the past, I was certain that someone had traveled from the initial hotspot with little or no symptoms and unknowingly spread the infection. In 2016, the world was racing to protect pregnant women and unborn children from Zika virus. In 2014, we were ramping up our infection protection protocols for the international spread of the

Ebola virus. In 2012, the Middle East Respiratory Syndrome, another novel Coronavirus, caused a worldwide panic. In each of these cases, the disease spread, but the travel cases were all identified and isolated, and the medical professionals and the scientific community worked together to prevent a pandemic.

January 24, 2020

The city of Wuhan is now on lockdown, but there are reports of people fleeing the city just before the lockdown. There are now cases of Coronavirus in Japan, Thailand, and South Korea. The US has a second case of Coronavirus, travel related, in Chicago. A buddy of mine is planning a trip with his wife to Bali in April. My wife and I were hoping to take our kids to Universal Studios this summer. At this point, I'm anticipating isolated cases to continue to pop up around the country, but nothing severe enough to disrupt future travel plans.

MYTH: Warm weather will kill the virus and stop the outbreak of Coronavirus.

Although the common cold and the flu viruses spread more during colder months and less in the summer, that is more about people spending more time in close proximity of each other and less about the actual air temperature. Currently, we do not know how warmer temperatures will affect the spread of COVID-19. It would be nice if it just disappeared into the sunset after winter ends, but I would not bet on it. Every virus has its own pattern of behavior based on its biochemical nature and we have not had enough time to learn what the pattern of the novel Coronavirus will be.

January 29, 2020

At this point, China is reporting about 2-3% mortality and we have 0 US deaths, so I'm thinking modern American medicine and infection control protocols are strong enough to protect us from this threat, just like it did with Ebola, SARS, and MERS. The strategy of early identification and isolation with detailed contact tracing has worked well in the past. My buddy who was going to Bali is rethinking his travel plans. The South China Sea is looking a bit unattractive right now. Looking toward the summer, I'm still thinking that we should be able to make our trip too.

Social media has discovered the word Coronavirus on the back of Lysol spray cans. They are now spreading conspiracies that we have nothing to fear because there isn't a new virus threatening our way of life and that everyone is overreacting. It's really scary how fast misinformation can spread. The Coronavirus family of viruses was first discovered over 50 years ago and is known for causing the common cold that people get every year. However, there have been other new members of this family that have recently caused international outbreaks, such as SARS and MERS. Although we do not have lab tested research proving that Lysol spray kills this novel Coronavirus, we fully expect that standard cleansing methods will kill the virus effectively.

MYTH: No one predicted another worldwide pandemic. No one could have seen this coming.

Intellectuals have been ringing alarm bells for years about how the world is not prepared for the next pandemic infection. Bill Gates of Microsoft gave a TED talk on the subject 5 years ago. No one talks about earthquakes as if there will never be another earthquake. No one talks about war as if there will never be another war. We watch and prepare and practice with drills for earthquakes and wars and now even active shooters. It was only a few short years ago we were facing the same situation initially with Ebola virus. Experts will tell you that we should have been preparing for the next pandemic as well.

Chapter 3

Outbreak

January 30, 2020

The World Health Organization has just declared Coronavirus a global health emergency after the US reported the first case of person-to-person transmission of the virus. On Fox News, some of the hosts speak dismissively about the severity of the virus and the scope of its spread. On CNN, the hosts are forecasting widespread doom and destruction. At this point, I feel like both are wrong. At least I hope so.

A guy at the store coughed ... I immediately wondered if he had Coronavirus. It didn't matter if he was old or young, brown or black or white ... he coughed ... and that worried me. Normally, I would hear a cough and not think twice, but now I hear a cough and I look both ways to find the culprit and secretly measure the distance between us. The fear that comes with this illness is surprising, a mix of the fear of the unknown and the fear of death.

There has been a lot of controversy about the use of facemasks since this outbreak started in China. For years, way before Coronavirus, people in major industrial cities of China have been wearing facemasks on a daily basis, not because of fear of an upcoming infection, but because of poor air quality. Search online and you will find images in China from years ago that look as though they belong to our current situation. Despite the widespread use of facemasks, Coronavirus spread to over 80,000 people in China and it will not completely protect you either.

MYTH: I should wear an N95 respiratory or surgical facemask and protect myself from Coronavirus

If a person with Coronavirus wears a facemask, the spread of infection may be reduced by the mask capturing the droplet particles that spread infection. Healthy individuals benefit when the ill wear a facemask. Similarly, screening individuals by measuring temperature offers community protection but does not offer individual protection. If a person has a fever because of Coronavirus, identifying that person may protect the future contacts of that person, but it does not offer any preventive benefit for the person with Coronavirus and fever. Proper hand washing remains the most effective method of preventing the infection. Please wash your hands for 20-30 seconds before touching your face or eating.

February 7, 2020

Li Wenliang, the Chinese doctor who was one of the first people to draw attention to the spread of Coronavirus, ended up getting the infection and passed away today. Without his actions to inform the public of the serious nature of this infection, the pandemic would likely be even worse.

The nearly 3000 people aboard the Diamond Princess cruise ship are still in quarantine off of the coast of Japan. A former passenger tested positive for Coronavirus on February 1 after spending 6 days on the ship. A few days later, 10 people tested positive. The Japanese authorities mandated a 14-day quarantine for all passengers while they confine themselves to their rooms.

February 15, 2020

African countries are being added to the travel ban ... but not because of Coronavirus. At this point there are no reported cases of COVID-19 in Africa. Travel to China has been limited, but the virus has already spread to the Middle East and Europe. There are 2 cases of Coronavirus in Italy. It seems like numbers rise in the places where they test more. In places where testing is limited, the numbers will remain low, but artificially. Soon, it will be unsafe to travel to any country, and the people traveling now to these places will undoubtedly continue to spread Coronavirus around the world.

MYTH: I should get a test for Coronavirus to prove that I am clean and so that I feel safe.

Every week I see patients who have been sent by their employer to get a Coronavirus test before returning to work. As a clinic manager, I understand the desire to maintain a safe workplace for all of the employees. Unfortunately, the limited supply of testing makes it nearly impossible for a person without signs of illness to get tested for Coronavirus. Currently, only the CDC is the only place conducting Coronavirus testing. The CDC sent out test kits to various labs around the country, but I have not heard from anyone that there is any local testing capability.

February 27, 2020

One of the patients who tested positive for COVID-19 in California had been hospitalized since February 19th and the physicians had been basically begging the CDC to authorize testing the patient but declined due to lack of travel history. I assume that proper precautions were taken while this patient was hospitalized, but what about all of the people who came into contact with this person before arriving at the hospital.

February 28, 2020

A second case of COVID-19 has been identified in California with no travel history. This suggests that someone else is walking around California with little or no symptoms of the virus and spreading it to others. Many viral infections have a phase of infection when the infected host has no symptoms and can still spread the virus, a phase of asymptomatic shedding. It would not be surprising if Coronavirus infection follows this pattern. If so, for every symptomatic Coronavirus infection, there may be 1 or 2 asymptomatic spreaders that we never detect.

There are some people who see the high-profile coverage of this infection and feel that the situation is overhyped. Some even feel that the infection is being used for political gain. By this point, the disease is spreading person to person within communities and we do not have testing to identify the infected, and therefore we cannot contain the spread of the infection. An illness that we cannot adequately test for that can spread before it causes symptoms is a troubling combination. You don't need to be a physician to predict what is happening. Common sense would tell you that this is going to get worse.

MYTH: Coronavirus is just like the flu (Influenza).

Half of my patients seem unconcerned about this outbreak, and the other half seem to take it very seriously. Although the flu does take thousands of lives every year, we have both a vaccine and anti-viral medications to help combat the disease. For Coronavirus, we don't have that. For some patients, symptoms of COVID-19 will feel similar to a case of the flu, but for others, the virus can cause severe damage to lung tissue, some of which may be long-lasting. Just like the flu, we cannot predict who gets a mild case and who gets a severe case. But, unlike the flu, if you get COVID-19, we have very few options to give you to help you recover faster. Combine that with the knowledge that the elderly has higher risk of death from COVID-19, and you arrive at the recommendation for the elderly to limit their social interactions as much as possible. The current numbers of cases and deaths from different countries show a mortality percentage rate similar to what we see each year with each flu season.

February 29, 2020

The first US patient has passed away from COVID-19. Italy has reported over a thousand cases of COVID-19 illnesses, but they still do not know how the outbreak started in Italy. The US begins to ban visitors who have traveled to China. US Citizens are exempt from this ban, but they will be "screened" upon arrival. Screening passengers from overseas for an illness that has no symptoms initially. Let's go back to the days after September 11, 2001 and pretend that the airport body scanners were very harmful to pregnant women. Well, the airport screeners would need a fast and reliable way to determine who is pregnant. Luckily, we have cheap, reliable, fast urine pregnancy tests. To effectively screen out Coronavirus, we would need a Coronavirus test of similar capabilities. Unfortunately, since we don't have anything like that, we will probably be unable to keep people with the virus out of our country.

March 2, 2020

One of the COVID-19 positive cruise ship passengers who was quarantined in San Antonio on the military base was released despite having a "weakly positive" third and final Coronavirus test. Although it's possible that this was just a testing error, the patient visited a local mall quite soon after release from the military base, which potentially could have exposed dozens or hundreds of people to Coronavirus. This also poses a different challenge. With flu season, we already know that a person can be sick with the flu and test negative for the flu. In the past, these patients would be misdiagnosed as having a cold, only to return in 1 or 2 days with worse symptoms and then test positive for the flu. We call this a false negative test, meaning that the test shows negative despite the patient having the disease. If the Coronavirus test can also have false-positive results, it could mean other people actually have the virus, test negative, and are actively mingling in the community instead of remaining in quarantine.

Water is disappearing from store shelves. So is toilet paper. Diarrhea is not a common symptom of coronavirus infection, but people sure are acting like it is. While staying well hydrated is good for your general health, there is no evidence that hydrating with hot liquids every 15 minutes will reduce the risk of infection from Coronavirus or any other infectious disease.

MYTH: Drinking sips of hot tea or hot water will wash Coronavirus down into your stomach and prevent you from getting the illness.

Heating food to temperatures above 180°F will likely kill most germs including COVID-19. Hot tea usually reaches similar temperatures but drinking hot liquids above 150°F can burn your oral surfaces without offering any significant benefit. Viral particles from respiratory droplets can enter the body from the nose as well as the mouth. Once inside, the virus likely enters the cells of the body quickly, which protects the virus from any high temperatures. Continuously drinking hot liquids will not raise the temperature of the internal cells or the respiratory tract high enough to kill any virus. Hydrate yourself in moderation, as overhydration can lead to electrolyte imbalances that can be dangerous.

March 4, 2020

Twenty-one people aboard the Grand Princess cruise ship have tested positive for the novel Coronavirus. I never really was fond of cruise ships, even before my first microbiology lecture on Norovirus, the gastrointestinal virus that causes severe diarrhea and is known to colonize cruise ships and cause frequent outbreaks. I always worried about getting sick on a cruise with no way off. Unfortunately, being on a ship with COVID-19 patients is definitely worse. The close quarters of a ship place additional risk of infection on all of the passengers. Proper quarantine would require a larger space so that passengers can isolate from each other and reduce risk of spread amongst each other.

Dr. Xavier Odili

The White House Coronavirus Task Force just announced that testing and treatment for Coronavirus will be categorized as an essential health benefit under the Affordable Care Act so that all insurance plans, private and public, including Medicare, must provide coverage for it. That's right, they are using Obamacare to mandate all insurance plans provide Coronavirus testing and treatment while they argue in court that Obamacare is unlawful and should be dissolved. I can't imagine how people will pay for healthcare if they lose their insurance during a crisis like this.

I just found out that one of my coworker's father passed away in January. His father was elderly and had pre-existing medical problems, but he was recovering and was transferred to a skilled nursing facility for rehab and conditioning. He was walking and breathing well on room air, but in less than a week, he developed a dry cough and found himself short of breath after walking. He soon needed supplemental oxygen and a chest x-ray revealed bilateral infiltrates suspicious for pneumonia. He was placed on a broad-spectrum antibiotic regimen and after 48 hours he was still getting worse. He was transferred to a hospital where he received multiple antibiotics. His chest x-ray did not improve, so a CT scan was performed and revealed bilateral ground-glass opacities, a pattern of lung damage that has also been seen in Coronavirus patients. His chest x-ray was normal 2 weeks before this. It made him wonder if he actually died from Coronavirus. In January, we weren't looking for COVID-19 in people who hadn't traveled, so there was no red flag raised. But, if people had been walking around with the virus with mild symptoms, it's possible that he may have received the virus from someone with minimal symptoms.

March 5, 2020

All my friends in health care are complaining about how difficult it is to order supplies now. Hospitals everywhere are stocking up and that is reducing supply inventory. Doctors across the country are experiencing similar difficulties. Stockpiles and inventory at some hospitals are at good levels, but the current level of use will deplete any size inventory because we are using so much more protective equipment because we are treating almost everyone as if they have the virus.

MYTH: Antivirals that work against the flu virus will work against Coronavirus.

There are new antivirals, such as Remdesivir, being developed that we hope will work against COVID-19. Labs are also testing existing antiviral drugs to see if any will have effect against Coronavirus. Unfortunately, none have been proven effective at this time. Patients with Coronavirus have been mistaken for Influenza patients and given Tamiflu and Xofluza, two antivirals effective against the flu, but the patients did not improve.

I keep reading reports of people breaking quarantine to attend public events. We know that it's hard to stay inside your home for two whole weeks, but people who have been asked to self-quarantine are risking the lives of so many others if they end up spreading the virus. If your health department or your doctor believes you are at increased risk to the general population, you are indirectly risking the health of your family and friends.

March 6, 2020

My friend who changed his Bali Trip to an England trip has now converted it to a Caribbean trip. The list of countries with no reports of cases is shrinking rapidly. So many people are infected around the world, I'm starting to wonder if this novel Coronavirus will become endemic in some countries and reoccur every year like the seasonal flu.

I help manage a clinic as medical director, which involves managing inventory of supplies. Lately, it has become nearly impossible to order N95 respirator masks. All our distributor options have the masks on backorder. The hospitals have priority on ordering them, and we have no estimate on when more will be available to clinics again. They say that people are buying the masks and hoarding them at home, which makes no sense if they haven't been fit-tested or taught how to properly wear it. Every day I see at least a dozen patients who are wearing simple surgical masks upside-down.

As much as everyone is relying on N95 respirator mask, no one talks about the actual filtering of the mask. Although there are several layers of fabric filtering the air, the size of the pores is between 100 and 300 nanometers wide, depending on the brand of N95 mask you have. Apparently, the diameter of the novel Coronavirus is about 125 nanometers. That technically means that Coronavirus particles could pass through the mask if given enough time. Despite that, the N95 mask provides exceptional form-fitting protection from outside particles. When properly sized and fitted, a person wearing an N95 respirator cannot smell any scents or fragrances, even if sprayed nearby. These are the main benefits the N95 mask offers over standard facemasks and the reasons why healthcare providers are in need of more.

March 8, 2020

Patients are asking for Coronavirus testing. They tell me that they heard on TV that anyone who wants a test can get a test. It's hard to tell them that no one in the city has testing except for the Harris County Health Department. People are scared and want reassurance about their health. Without treatment or vaccine, they are asking for all that's left. In truth, if a patient with mild symptoms were to test positive, that patient would be discharged home and given precautions to isolate at home for a minimum of 14 days.
If we had an adequate supply of tests, we might be able to test all COVID-19 patients after 7 days or 10 days and discover a shorter healing time, but even with better data,

there would always be individuals who experience symptoms outside of the normal timeframe.

MYTH: Everyone who wants a test for COVID-19 should get a test.

In general, most tests must be ordered by a physician after he or she examines you and discusses your symptoms with you. Given the limited supply of testing for COVID-19, making sure tests are used appropriately is even more important. As a physician, I understand why people are worried and why they want to be tested, but we must reserve tests for the situations that make the most clinical impact. A person with mild fever and light cough can isolate at home unless symptoms worsen, leaving testing available for patients requiring critical care. Eventually, more tests will be available, and more people will be able to get tested.

March 9, 2020

Over half a dozen Houstonians returning from Egypt have all tested positive for Coronavirus, with even more people under suspicion. Interestingly enough, there are no reports at this time of large outbreaks in Egypt. There was a delay in identifying these individuals because it takes times for symptoms to appear, but there was certainly public exposure while each of these persons was continuing with daily life activities. In about 2 weeks, we should expect to see a sharp rise in the number of COVID-19 cases in the

Greater Houston area ... if we have an adequate supply of tests by then.

The entire country of Italy is now asked to stay home as much as possible, a country-wide lockdown. It's definitely the right move given the rapid spread of Coronavirus in their country. It will take a while to see the benefits though, because the virus has a variable incubation period. This means that it can lay dormant in your body from 2 to 14 days before manifesting symptoms. Because of this long incubation period, suspected contacts are advised that they must wait 14 days before testing negative and release.

A member of the US House of Representatives is self-quarantined at home after exposure to a COVID-19 positive patient, the same Representative who wore a gas mask as he voted against the first relief bill to help Americans by increasing funding for the CDC. Luckily, the bill passed because nearly everyone else in Congress voted for the bill. It's not a good look to make fun of a situation that is impacting the lives of so many people around the world.

March 10, 2020

No vaccine, no antivirals, no effective treatment ... and now reports of patients getting clear of the infection, testing negative, and then getting infected again ... if acquired immunity after infection doesn't last long, it's possible that people could get infected again. Every year I see patients who get Influenza infections twice in the same season. All the more reason to practice proper hand hygiene and social distancing. You literally should be protecting yourself as if everyone else has Coronavirus.

MYTH: Only the elderly is at risk of death or severe illness from Coronavirus.

Because COVID-19 is a novel or new strain of Coronavirus, we do not expect any age group to be immune from infection. This means that everyone is at risk of infection and that outcomes will vary person to person. Data from China showed that patients 70 and above suffered worse outcomes and a higher death rates, but data from Italy reveal that hospitalized patients between the ages of 20 and 45 make up about 25% of the country's cases of COVID-19 infection. Hospitals in Italy report that about half of their hospitalized patients are under the age of 65, many below the age of 45. In the US, we have also seen significant numbers of people between the ages 20 and 45 fall ill because of COVID-19.

A coworker recently died, an ER nurse. She tested positive for Influenza and took Tamiflu. She continued to work while she thought she was recovering. Unfortunately, she died in her sleep, reportedly from cardiac complications of Influenza infection. Although the US did not have Coronavirus testing at the time she passed away, we assumed that the Influenza was the only infection in her system. Tens of thousands of people die from the flu every year, people of varying ages. Despite this fact, every year only a fraction of the US population receives the flu vaccine. Every year I have to convince parents to use Tamiflu to treat their flu-test-positive children. They hesitate because of risk of side effects and rare reports of negative effects of Tamiflu. The flu kills so many people each year and we still have to work so hard to get people to use vaccines and antivirals to save lives. It makes me wonder if it would be different if we had a vaccine or an antiviral treatment for Coronavirus.

Chapter 4

Containing the Contagion

March 11, 2020

The World Health Organization has officially declared the Coronavirus outbreak a global pandemic. There are over 120,000 cases worldwide and over 1200 cases here in the United States. The US government has suspended travel to Europe after COVID-19 cases and deaths spike in Italy and the NBA cancels games after a Utah Jazz player tests positive for COVID-19. Tom Hanks also tests positive, and people are starting to wonder how the rich and famous are getting tested and results so quickly when doctors all around the country are struggling to get tests for sick patients.

The Houston Rodeo finally cancelled the rest of the shows after the city found out that a COVID-19 positive patient attended the BBQ Cook-Off the previous week. Austin cancelled South by Southwest a week ago, but it was definitely the right decision. We already know that it takes something like a full city shut down to prevent the illness from spreading. Having a large-scale event where people mingle and interact was tempting fate at best and most likely putting the public in unnecessary danger.

My oldest son is shocked that the NBA has cancelled the remainder of the season. He's a big fan of Zion. Earlier he was debating with his grandmother about which virus was worse, Coronavirus or Influenza. He had done his homework and already knew that the flu kills tens of thousands every year. I told him that we don't really know how bad this outbreak is going to be. Then I told him that the NBA season was cancelled ... he was speechless.

A friend of mine just got back from Colombia and said that there is no Coronavirus hysteria there. Restaurants and hotels were open, and stores fully stocked. Meanwhile, in the US, the hoarding is in full effect. Someone's garage must have a really tall tower of toilet paper and water bottles right now. People in this city are starting to panic, and this is going on with minimal testing capacity. Once we are able to test a larger portion of the population, we will actually be able to get a clear picture of just how many people in the city have Coronavirus. It may sound reassuring that only a small number of people test positive for disease, but only when a large number of people have been tested. If the number of persons tested is small as well, a low infection rate can be misleading at best and possibly lead to future misguided actions or decisions.

March 12, 2020

School districts in the area are all announcing they will remain closed for an additional 1-2 weeks after Spring Break to help slow the spread of Coronavirus. Looking at China's numbers and seeing that the city of Wuhan has been on lockdown for almost 2 months and they are still reporting new cases and deaths, I can already see that 2 weeks of school closure is not going to be enough. I tell my wife that we should prepare to not go back to school for the rest of this school year.

MYTH: Airport screening measures will prevent any COVID-19 carriers from coming into the US.

Europe travel ban has been clarified and does not include the UK. Coronavirus cases and deaths are rising all over Europe, so I don't see how someone would feel comfortable with one country and worried about another. Coronavirus crossed the Pacific Ocean, so I'm sure it's crossing the English Channel too. No matter how many temperature checks and questionnaires they give to people as they board or walk off the plane, there will be people, both American and visitors, who will be carrying the Coronavirus and showing no symptoms. Without rapid testing, there can be no perfect screening measures.

Worldwide there are over 145,000 cases of Coronavirus, and in the US, there are over 1600 cases of Coronavirus infection. After the NBA suspended its season, the NHL,

MLS, Tennis, and even international soccer suspended current play. I guess it's only a matter of time before the Olympics postpones as well. I don't see a way forward for any form of contact sports while we know so little about this virus.

March 13, 2020

Before Coronavirus, I would tell patients that they should consider staying home if they feel sick so that they don't expose others to illness unnecessarily. A passenger on JetBlue notified the crew that he was COVID-19 positive at the end of the flight after landing. He wore a surgical facemask the entire flight and sat across the aisle from his wife. Luckily no one was sitting next to him, but I'm sure that no one on that plane is going to have a good night's sleep for a while.

Americans have been rushing back to the US ahead of the planned start date for the Europe travel ban. If international visitors are banned from coming, those flight will start to get cut. My neighbor tells me that they paid over a thousand dollars to bring back their daughter who was in Europe for Spring Break. I can only imagine the crowds at the airport when these packed flights return. If anyone coming back did have Coronavirus, they would be forced into waiting in long lines of customs or a crowd of people waiting to get through the process, increasing the risk to everyone around them.

I'm hearing that turnaround time on COVID-19 testing is 3-4 days with Harris County. That seems so long when you are trying to separate them from the general public to reduce risk of spread. In other countries, testing is much more rapid and robust, allowing for better identification and isolation of Coronavirus patients. Here, I feel like the patients are right in front of us, but we can't identify them from the other respiratory illness patients.

Never have I ever seen so much news coverage on Fox News. I have been watching Fox News since about 2015 and it's usually split 60/40 between news coverage and opinion shows. At some point, they must have had a big morning meeting to tell everyone to cease and desist with the hoax talk, but a couple of people missed that meeting. They continued to refer to the worldwide spread of this infection as a hoax and were quickly replaced with real journalists reporting real news. If I didn't already know how serious this all is, I do now.

March 14, 2020

A coworker just told me that the UK Health Minister has announced that their plan to combat the Coronavirus epidemic is herd immunity. I literally laughed out loud. Herd immunity is the name for the situation where a group of people have protection from a threat, although individually, not everyone in the herd has protection. Think of a herd of gazelle in the wild. A single gazelle has little defense against a lion or other dangerous predator.

However, a herd of gazelle pose a more difficult target to most predators. The very young and elderly of the herd are usually protected at the center and the stronger adults less likely to fall prey form the outer barrier.

With infections, we usually use vaccines to create immunity, but we know that infants are not born immune and do not receive enough vaccine to prevent infection for many months. During that time, we rely on the immunity of everyone else to shield the young from infection. Not everyone has to be vaccinated to keep the population free from disease, but a large percentage of the population needs that immunity for everyone to benefit.

MYTH: Herd immunity is a safe way to protect everyone from Coronavirus.

If you try to apply the concept of herd immunity to a population with no immunity and no vaccine, you then will have to wait for people to develop immunity after being infected. This means that the UK Health Minister was proposing the plan of defense against the virus was to let everyone (or almost everyone) get the virus and then, eventually, develop immunity ... if they survived. To purposefully plan for the population to get sick is the same as planning for a percentage of those people to die. All methods of prevention would be preferable to waiting for herd immunity.

Dr. Xavier Odili

March 15, 2020

The CDC has recommended that school closures for 8 weeks or longer may be needed to sufficiently slow the spread of Coronavirus. They also recommend against gatherings of 50 or more people. These steps are going in the right direction. Eliminating hugs and handshakes and reinforcing proper handwashing techniques are all part of the steps needed to prevent a healthcare crisis in this country.

MYTH: Lysol spray will kill Coronavirus in midair.

It's understandable that everyone wants to do everything they can to protect themselves, but I have to say that I am tired of walking into a room and breathing in from a cloud of Lysol Disinfectant Spray. The instructions on the can clearly state exactly which types of surfaces can be cleansed with the spray. That's right ... surfaces. Hard surfaces, soft surfaces, semi-porous surfaces ... but nothing about killing anything in the air. After spraying onto your surface of choice, it is equally important to let the spray stand for the necessary amount of time to completely kill the germs. Wiping the Lysol away does not kill the germs. The amount of time you are instructed to wait depends on the germs you are intending to kill. Most germs are killed in 2 minutes, but some require ten minutes. This means you need to spray and walk away if you want to use Lysol correctly.

The ER Physician Facebook group I follow is full of stories from physicians telling how their hospitals are low on protective equipment like gowns and N95 respirators. Several are having to reuse masks day after day. Right now, hospitals in Italy are overwhelmed with sick patients. In some cities, doctors have run out of critical care beds and ventilators and literally have to decide which patients get ventilators and live, and which patients do not.

March 16, 2020

Patients keep sounding surprised that we are seeing cases of COVID-19 in their vicinity. There must not be enough reporters to report everything that is going on. The call for social distancing isn't settling in very well. I get the sense that some people feel like Coronavirus is still an "out there" problem and not a local problem. I'm sure that this is partly due to a lack of local testing but also partly due to confidentiality of medical testing. Hospital systems are not publicizing the number of patients they have, so people are unaware of how widespread the infection has become.

MYTH: People of Asian descent are more likely to carry or have Coronavirus.

I heard that there was an overseas rumor that the US military brought the Coronavirus to China to infect them. Soon after, I started hearing US officials calling COVID-19 the "Chinese Virus" or the "Kung Flu". Although this particular virus was first reported in China, we never blame the country of origin or its people. Disease outbreaks have come from all parts of the world and from all types of vectors. Just a few months ago we were telling people to avoid putting hard boiled eggs on salads. Before that, there was an outbreak of diarrhea and vomiting symptoms that was traced back to romaine lettuce. Years ago, a different strain of Coronavirus originated in the Middle East and caused severe illness they called Middle East Respiratory Syndrome. Ten years ago, a new variation of the flu jumped from pigs to humans and caused the Swine Flu epidemic. Decades ago, we were worried about Mad Cow Disease and China was refusing to purchase American beef products. Disease happens, and we all need to work together to get through them, not point fingers and lay blame upon one another.

Disneyland, Disney World, and Universal Studios have closed the doors to their theme parks and attractions. The way this virus spreads, it would not be surprising if every major venue closed, whether the government mandates it or not. Several of my neighbors are home now as well. They ask if the clinic will close or stay open and if we test for Coronavirus. Because of the shortage of testing equipment and the guidance to use the tests for only the hospitalized, we are not testing for COVID-19. It would be good to be able to test people and provide reassurance to people, but even if we had tests, we do not have adequate supply of protective equipment to handle the amount of people we would expect to come in if we did offer tests.

March 17, 2020

The CDC has now recommended no gatherings of more than 10 people. This is moving closer and closer to the home isolation strategy that seems to be working in China. In Europe, they are struggling with social distancing and home isolation. In the coming weeks, we will see if our efforts were sufficient enough to "flatten the curve" and slow the spread of infection to a level where our hospital systems can handle the numbers of sick patients without having to open up temporary care units and field hospitals.

The first human trials of the Coronavirus vaccine have started. This round of testing is a safety test, which involves giving the vaccine to healthy individuals to see if they have any side effects or complications. Thank you to the brave individuals who volunteered for this trial. After several weeks or months of monitoring them for side effects and unexpected symptoms, we hope that the safety of the vaccine will be verified. The next step would be a clinical trial to test the effectiveness of the vaccine to prevent people from getting Coronavirus. Hopefully, by next year we will have an approved vaccine that we can use to help in the future.

MYTH: The Coronavirus vaccine will be ready for the public in a few weeks.

The number of cases in New York is growing exponentially. Honestly, I'm impressed that they have that many tests. I've lived in New York and I know first-hand how dense the city is, so I'm not surprised the virus is spreading like wildfire. Subways are like sardine cans. People jam pack on elevators. Are cabs even cleaned between passengers? My sister works in NYC in Urgent Care and she is seeing people sick enough to transfer to the hospital by EMS with negative flu tests. She tells me that she has proper protective equipment, but I still pray for her safety.

A mom came in today with her grandmother carrying a toddler in her arms. Just prior to arrival, they were playing in the bedroom and jumping on the bed. He landed in a bad way and has not been able to stand up since the fall. I examined him, and in less than a minute I could tell that his femur was fractured. The x-ray confirmed it, and we transferred the patient for Pediatric Orthopedics consultation. Every now and then, someone will ask me if it's worth it … is it worth the risk to me, my wife, my kids to be on the front lines providing care when the risks today seem higher than ever before. Every day we make a difference in the lives of our patients and their families, and we are not going to let Coronavirus stop us.

March 18, 2020

Patients keep asking about Coronavirus testing, which is understandable. It's so hard to tell them that the disease is spreading, and the County has all the tests and even if they go to the hospital with symptoms, they probably will not be able to get tested. The city was hoping to open up drive thru testing centers for the public, but they have delayed that opening.

The Health Department called to tell us that one of our patients tested positive for COVID-19. I saw the caller ID and time slowed down while my heart sped up. I know that every day I work, I risk myself contracting an illness, not just Coronavirus, but Influenza or another respiratory virus. I usually get the flu every year or every other year, even though I get the flu vaccine. When I get it, I usually quarantine myself for a few days and sleep in the closet. I take my medicine, and I feel back to normal a few days later, and I have never passed the flu on to my family. As bad as the flu makes you feel, I would feel even worse if my family got it from me. I couldn't live with myself if I brought Coronavirus home.

I keep hearing people say this is an invisible enemy. Well, it wouldn't be invisible if we had adequate testing. I don't mean testing that takes 3-4 days for a result, but same day testing, or at least within 24 hours. Two military hospital ships are supposed to be dispatched to provide assistance to New York and also to the West Coast hotspots. I appreciate the willingness of our military to follow orders and rush into harm's way for the good of the American people. However, without widespread testing with rapid results, people with mild symptoms will carry Coronavirus onto the medical ships in the same way they carried it onto cruise ships.

Dr. Xavier Odili

March 19, 2020

My coworkers now all have stories of seeing COVID-19 positive patients, but because of the lack of tests, they are all hearing about it many days after exposure. We are starting to see fewer non-emergency patients in the ER. Maybe people are worried about the risk of sitting in a waiting room of strangers and leaving with a problem worse than the reason you initially came for. That risk has always existed, but it just seems more real these days.

Yesterday, the US and Canada "closed" its border to non-essential travel but not goods and trade ... I'm not sure if the US is worried about infected people sneaking in or if Canada was worried about the infection in Washington state and New York state spreading into Canada.

FDA reports it's working on approving Chloroquine for use to treat Coronavirus, based on success in a few cases. As a people, we need rays of hope to guide us forward as we continue this journey. As a physician, I realize that we do not have the evidence to say with certainty that this old drug that has been used for treating Malaria for years will have any reliable and consistent effect on patients with Coronavirus. Hopefully, clinical trials are being designed so that we can find out how effective it could be.

Apparently, Governors have asked for the US government to assist with procuring ventilators, but they have been told that they are responsible for getting their own ventilators to fill any shortages they have. Imagine if you have a shortage of toilet paper and 50 people need it ... those people are going to offer more money to get what they need and that drives up the price of the product. If all of the states are bidding for the same ventilators, that makes the price higher than it would be if the US government brokered the deal and secured a set price for everyone. Which option seems more sensible to you? We need a single purchaser to negotiate the best deal for everyone.

MYTH: "Flattening the curve" means that we reduce the number of cases of infection and we return to normal life faster.

We have learned from the past that when an infection outbreak occurs, without any intervention, the infection will spread faster and faster, rising exponentially until a majority of the population is infected. By the time that happens, there are not many people left to get infected anymore, so the number of infections start to fall until there are no more people left to infect. Unfortunately, if illnesses rise too quickly, the hospitals will be overwhelmed and unable to handle the number of people who will need medical care. To "flatten the curve" means to slow down that rapid rise and spread out the infections over a much longer time period so that when people get sick, the hospitals are able to keep up with the demand for hospital treatment.

March 20, 2020

Last night the Governor of California placed the entire state on "shelter in place" and this morning, the Governor of New York did the same thing for all the people in that state. I think that this is the right thing to do and a good time to do it. It would have been better if it happened sooner, but I know that it would have been very hard for people to adjust to such a drastic change in way of life. We know that in Wuhan, China, similar lockdown measures were implemented and after several weeks, the reported number of new cases has fallen all the way down to zero. However, this data may not be reliable, as China's government has withheld or manipulated statistics about their country in the past. Still, I worry about what happens when people return to normal mingling and movement ... will the virus re-emerge? Without a robust method of identifying the ill and contacting the casual contacts of the ill, how can any country hope to contain such a contagious disease?

The US Border with Mexico has now closed for non-essential person travel ... I understand the use of a multifaceted approach which is using everything possible to reduce the spread of the virus. Restricting travel is just as important as social distancing. I still feel sad that we don't have enough tests to properly identify the carriers of this virus and properly limit spread instead of these secondary and tertiary measures. Although people traveling from other countries might be carrying the disease, citizens who live here now are carrying the disease in plain sight.

MYTH: If I don't have fever or cough, I probably don't have Coronavirus.

A local man in his 30s walked in 2 weeks ago with sudden onset body aches and chills, but no fever or cough or sore throat. He was diagnosed and treated for the flu and proceeded to travel out of state by commercial airplane with his family for Spring Break vacation. While in Florida, his symptoms worsened. He had planned to visit the major theme parks, which had not yet closed, but he felt so ill that he had to stay in the hotel room. The same day he flew back to Houston, he returned to our clinic in worse condition, with fever, rapid heart rate, and low blood pressure. He was transferred to a local hospital for evaluation and 3 days later, tested positive for COVID-19. This patient unknowingly exposed Coronavirus to his family, friends, coworkers, and the strangers he shared a plane or cab or airport shuttle with, as well as the healthcare workers who cared for him.

Literally anyone could have Coronavirus, and people are walking around and sharing it with others without even knowing it. A rapid test may have helped prevent much of this unnecessary spread, but for now, we must approach this with isolation and common sense. If you feel sick, you should stay home until you feel better. Isolate yourself from people as much as possible. Call your doctor's office and explain your symptoms and ask for a work excuse. Many offices are using telemedicine to have visits with patients from the safety of their own home.

Cases doubled overnight in New York and deaths in Italy surpassed deaths in China. Houston finally has it's drive thru testing up and running and one of my colleagues went to get tested. Another coworker went and was denied testing. Both were exposed to the same COVID-19 positive patient. Apparently, the system isn't ready to test all who need a test, which is frustrating because we can't ever get ahead of this if we can't identify who has it.

Iran is now publicly calling for investigation of the US for spreading COVID-19 to China and Iran. This reminds me of nearly every young couple who both test positive for an STD - each side blames the other for giving them the disease.

March 21, 2020

There have been daily briefings from the US Coronavirus Task Force for over a week now. It seems weird that I get my updates on government policy regarding this pandemic from a daily televised briefing. These updates are different from the conference calls and meetings I have almost every day locally and the information discussed is different. In one, I am hearing the government overview of how the system will be designed for the country to combat this threat. In the other, I get the "boots on the ground" marching orders from my Head of Department. Both sets of information are necessary to formulate a successful plan of action.

People are talking about the combination of Hydroxychloroquine and Azithromycin as possible treatment for Coronavirus, but I haven't seen any formal recommendation from the FDA or heard about any colleagues using the combo. Chloroquine and Hydroxychloroquine have been used for decades in preventing or treating malaria and in treating lupus and rheumatoid arthritis. Evidence-based medicine means using evidence from research or clinical trials to guide your practice of medicine. Treating people based on a hunch or what worked in one or two places outside of the country is not consistent with evidence-based medicine and best practices. I expect that in the next two weeks, we will see if this combination is effective at saving lives here at home. Further study is needed to determine important details of how the medicine should best be used, such as dose, frequency, and duration. A hammer is a good tool for driving in nails, but it is not a good tool for removing teeth. We know that these medicines are useful in the daily management of lupus and other arthritic diseases, and to preserve the supply of this medicine for everyone who needs it, we should allow researchers to continue to determine the lowest dose that is most effective in treatment.

We have evidence from other countries that the combination of Hydroxychloroquine and Azithromycin has been shown to be effective in reducing the amount of virus in hospitalized patients, leading to faster recovery in those patients. We do not have information on how the medicine affects people who are not yet critically ill. We also have no idea if it would be effective in preventing people from getting Coronavirus. If it can be used to reduce risk of getting infected, we will finally have a new tool in slowing the spread of the infection. If not, we are looking at several more weeks of this infection spreading.

Essentially, we have to assume that every patient has COVID-19 and protect ourselves from every patient. Even if we had instant testing, in the Emergency Department and in Urgent Care, we would still behave the same way because symptoms vary so much that we can't easily identify likely suspects. Our initial contact with the patient is the most dangerous because we know nothing about the patient until we spend time to ask the important questions. Because doctors and nurses have to use the appropriate protection for almost every patient, we are using much more protective equipment each day than ever before.

The city of Houston is reporting over 100 cases now. I don't know if this is because the drive-up testing numbers are being released or if this is just from tests performed in hospitals. Up until now, only patients being admitted to hospitals are getting tested for COVID-19, not emergency room patients who are discharged home because they are not severely ill. The CDC is now advising a similar policy for testing across the country, to preserve the supply of tests for the hospitalized patients.

The New York governor is painting a very bleak picture. A worldwide illness has increased demand and the increase in sick patients has reduced the supply. It's good that companies are switching from making liquor to hand sanitizer and converting other manufacturing plants to be able to manufacture masks and gowns and gloves because we're going to need them.

March 22, 2020

I just listened to an interview of one of the ER doctors from Kirkland, Washington, the city near Seattle where COVID-19 was first identified. It was great to hear his thoughts about their experience. He corroborated some things that we already knew from 2 months ago, that people were getting sick with COVID-19 that had not traveled anywhere, and the testing criteria mandated by the CDC was so strict that they were not able to get tests for the patients they were suspecting. It wasn't until the testing criteria were relaxed that they were able to confirm their suspicions. You have no idea how dangerous that is. Imagine every large and moderate city in America experiencing an outbreak like Seattle. We do not have enough supply of protective equipment to handle every single patient in every hospital in every city like they are carrying Coronavirus. To use our supplies wisely so that they do not run out, we must be able to identify and separate Coronavirus patients from those who test negative.

MYTH: After 2 weeks of home isolation and social distancing, the virus will die off and life can return to normal.

I've been on a conference call with the hospital group I work with every day or every other day to talk about logistics and citywide overview of how the infection is spreading. We are living in the calm before the storm. We are all hoping that the storm never comes, but we are preparing for it to be as bad as what we are seeing in New York City. We are all preparing for a months-long battle against Coronavirus. We hope to see a slow rise in the number of infected persons, which would be proof that social distancing is working. If people ignore these recommendations, the virus will continue to spread, and hospitals will be overwhelmed with seriously ill patients.

The struggle is real. It's hard to adjust to this new kind of life. It's one thing to ask adults to adjust to a life of social distancing. It's hard to get kids to understand and nearly impossible for toddlers to understand. Today makes 2 weeks straight with all the kids at home because school is closed, and we pulled the little ones out of daycare. The kids miss their teachers and friends. My wife is getting cabin fever. Because I work 6 days a week, I also try to do the shopping while I'm out. I also didn't feel comfortable with her going to the store and possibly being exposed, and to me, shopping with the general public is probably just as risky as working a shift in the ER.

Cities across the country are applying social distancing across all aspects of life. Convention centers and homeless shelters are closing. They have also been releasing low-level criminal offenders to avoid a prison outbreak of Coronavirus. The news is reporting that Harvey Weinstein tested positive for COVID-19. I'm just shocked that doctors around the country are struggling to get sick patients tested and celebrities seem to have no problem, but hey, celebrities are people too. The fear of the unknown is real and everyone is susceptible to it.

March 23, 2020

Over 35,000 cases of Coronavirus in America at this point. National Guard is setting up much-needed mobile hospitals in New York, California, and Washington. A new type of Coronavirus test is pending approval and claims to report results in under an hour. A rapid and reliable test is needed for many reasons. Without rapid testing, we are not able to tell if people arriving from international travel are carrying the virus. Without rapid testing, the staff of the military hospital ships heading to the east and west coasts will be unable to ensure that they are not letting infected patients aboard the ships. Even the White House can't be sure that reporters and visitors who enter on a daily basis are free of infection without rapid testing. But most importantly, healthcare providers can't make quick decisions about their patients without rapid testing. With so many new types of potential treatments on the horizon, we need adequate testing to decide who should even get the new treatments.

Dr. Xavier Odili

MYTH: The ER will test me for Coronavirus if I have traveled out of the US or if I am concerned about being infected with Coronavirus.

My neighbor took a little fall today and injured his foot. He works for a major hospital system in Houston and even though he was worried he has a fracture, he is afraid to go to the ER for evaluation. The threat of Coronavirus is so real that even people who work at the hospital are unwilling to take the risk of sitting in an emergency room lobby and potentially be exposed to someone carrying the virus. Due to the lack of adequate testing availability, recommendations from several areas of government and medical leadership are all in agreement. Tests should be saved for patients needing hospitalization. It is highly unlikely that a hospital ER will use a test on someone who is destined to go back home, no matter how concerned that person may be. At some point in the future, we hope to have enough tests to test everyone who wants a test.

Evening news reports the number of cases has risen to over 42000. Nearly 550 people have lost their lives. 14 different Governors have issued stay at home orders to their states, and people are still talking about resuming business as usual in a week. I just don't see it. The train has left the station folks, and it's still picking up steam. We are nowhere near the peak of this and there are no brakes to stop it.

Meanwhile, in South Korea, an aggressive approach to widespread testing and high-tech monitoring has successfully slowed down the spread of Coronavirus. By setting up over 500 testing sites across the country very early on in the outbreak, and using cell phone GPS tracking systems, the authorities of South Korea were able to isolate everyone who needed to be isolated and slow down the rate of increase of infections. No hospitals in South Korea were overwhelmed by patients. No healthcare providers ran out of any medical protective equipment. Early testing and isolation combined school closures, social distancing, and travel restrictions saved the country.

March 24, 2020

UK Prime Minister Boris Johnson has issued strict stay at home orders for the entire country. I'm so relieved they are doing more than just waiting for enough people to get sick and eventually develop herd immunity. Italy reports another 746 deaths today. A number of different trackers show that US numbers have consistently been about 10 days behind Italy numbers. Our only hope of avoiding that future is to be very aggressive with our social distancing and staying at home.

Governor Cuomo of New York reports that cases of COVID-19 are doubling every 3 days. New York has spent a little over a week under strict "Stay at Home" orders, but due to the long incubation period of Coronavirus, they will not be able to hope to see a difference for a minimum of 2 weeks. It's probably true that the stay at home orders were given after the virus had spread significantly and the best outcome, they can hope for is a "flattening of the curve" and a slowing of the sharp rise of cases and deaths.

Harris County has issued a stay at home order for the general public with some exceptions to last about 10 days. Although some people are optimistic that we will be able to resume normal life in the next 2 weeks, history has shown us that illness takes longer to rise and fall. Furthermore, if our efforts to slow the spread are effective, we will be extending the length of the illness moving through our society even longer.

MYTH: Children and young people are immune to the effects of Coronavirus.

Today, California authorities reported that a teenager passed away due to complications from COVID-19 infection, the first child to die in the US from Coronavirus. In Georgia, a 12-year-old child has been placed on a ventilator to assist with breathing due to lung damage from Coronavirus. Studies evaluating COVID-19 hospitalized patients in the US show 20% of hospitalized cases involve patients between the ages of 20 and 44. Children and young people can be severely affected by this virus. No one is immune.

President Xi of China has reported plans to relax the restrictions on the people living in Wuhan in the days to come. This will be the world's first test of how the infection will proceed after a prolonged social distancing and stay at home enforcement. For months, the people have been in isolation and the number of daily new cases of infection has been falling, and recently was reported no new cases. If all of the people with infection remain in isolation, the people resuming normal life should have little risk of getting or spreading Coronavirus. If their plans are successful, the whole world will have hope for a bright future on the other side of this pandemic.

March 25, 2020

The US now has over 60,000 cases of COVID-19 and over 800 deaths. More and more stories from different parts of the country reveal the severe shortages in ability to handle the sharp rise in sick patients. New Jersey and Louisiana seem to be right behind New York in terms of rapid rise of cases of infection. People in different parts of the country might be wondering if Coronavirus is going to reach them. It's not a matter of if, but when.

Doctors, nurses, and healthcare providers in Italy are dying from COVID-19, partly due to lack of protective equipment and partly due to the highly contagious nature of this virus. We do not have enough tests to find all of the people who have Coronavirus in the US, and every day that an infected person is out and about, 2 to 4 more people are probably contracting the virus. The only tool we have to slow down this spread is social distancing, and even if we perform that to the maximum, it will still spread because there are parts of our society that require close contact. If we do not take this seriously, cases may continue to rise until the disease no longer has healthy people to infect.

The FDA is working to approve the use of convalescent plasma immune therapy for treatment of COVID-19 patients. People who were infected with COVID-19 and recovered from their infection have developed antibodies that would protect their body from the infection coming back. The idea is that if we get a sufficient supply of these antibodies from the recovered patients, we could then inject the antibodies into current patients to help them fight their current infection. This type of treatment is called passive antibody therapy and it has been effective at reducing the severity of illness with patients infected with SARS and Ebola viruses in the past. Currently there is not a large number of recovered patients, so there is not enough raw material to treat all the people who may need it. There is also no evidence that this type of immunity would be effective as a vaccine. Still, it is another potential weapon we can use to prevent people from dying.

March 26, 2020

The death toll from COVID-19 in the US has passed 1000 today. Some people are comparing this to the impact of Influenza, which kills 10,000 to 20,000 people or more each year. After 2 months of illness, it would be hard to make any comparison. All of the tracking charts show that the rate of infection is still going up. We are at the point that so many people are sick with this virus that we may not be able to eradicate it. It's possible that a majority of the country may eventually get this disease, whether it's this year or next or the year after that.

A patient called today. He has been having cough and congestion and had recently returned from travel out of state. He wanted to know if it was safe for him to come into clinic for an evaluation. His symptoms and travel were definitely concerning for Coronavirus, and it was not safe for us or the other patients in our clinic for him to come in. Thanks to telemedicine, we can initiate visits over the internet and reduce the risk of spreading infection.

Coworkers keep telling me about their friends and family are convinced that this is a hoax, that the threat isn't real, that the burden of illness is being hyped up, and that we are all overreacting. To be clear, real hospitals are converting outpatient areas and standard care areas into ICU critical care space to take care of real patients who are really sick. In New York, healthcare providers are telling their stories and their needs are real. The US now has the second highest total number of Coronavirus infection cases in the world, second only to China, and by the end of the week the US will have the most cases of any country in the world. Over 230 Americans have died due to Coronavirus infection today, a majority in New York, the deadliest day of this pandemic so far. If we as a nation are not able to provide supplies and support for one city that hasn't even reached the peak of illness, what are we going to do when there are multiple cities facing the same threats?

We have entered a new age, one without sports to distract us or travel to relax us. A new age where we must lean on our family and neighbors and friends for support. When faced with uncertainty, they say that physicians don't panic, we prepare. The fight against Coronavirus is going to be a marathon, not a sprint.

Chapter 5

Leading the World

March 27, 2020

The US now leads the world in total number of cases of Coronavirus infection, now over 90,000 cases, with no signs of slowing down. Hospitals in cities across the country are filling with patient. In Europe, there continue to be increasing numbers of death and infection, and now reports from African nations indicate rapid spread. In Italy, the death toll for today alone is nearly 1000 people. By the end of the day we will have more than 100,000 cases in the US. Nearly half of those cases will be in the New York area. I suspect that the rapid spread of disease in New York may be related to how densely packed the population is and perhaps even the use of public transportation. The compact nature of the city is very close in character to European cities, where rapid rise in infection has been reported for weeks. Only time will tell, but this is just another reason to avoid crowded spaces and continue social distancing.

First responders and health care providers are falling ill as they man the front lines against this pandemic. Personal protective equipment is fundamental to the success of this battle, but so are ventilators. Fortunately, General Motors has announced that it will begin manufacturing ventilators.

But why do we need so many ventilators? Typically, a person with Coronavirus would need to cough or sneeze to release droplet particles of infection into the air. When a patient is having difficulty breathing, normally, we would offer a nebulizer breathing treatment or high flow oxygen to help. Unfortunately, these treatment options actually disperse large amounts of tiny respiratory droplets into the air surrounding the patient, which exposes the healthcare providers to even greater risk of getting Coronavirus. Without those usual options, we only have one option left for a patient who is having trouble breathing … we must intubate and place a breathing tube which then must be connected to a ventilator. Essentially, we need a minimum of 2 to 3 times as many ventilators at every hospital above the normal amount to account for the increase number of anticipated intubations.

MYTH: Getting a Coronavirus infection is an automatic death sentence.

Although there have been thousands of people who lost their lives to COVID-19, hundreds of thousands of people survive. Even without specific prescription treatment, this is definitely not an automatic death sentence. You may be shocked to hear how professional athletes and movie stars are getting infected. Even the UK Prime Minister has reported that he has tested positive for COVID-19, Prince Charles of the British Royal Family reported having the infection last week. And yet, there is hope. A 90-year-old woman in Kirkland near Seattle, Washington has recovered after falling ill with COVID-19. In Italy, a 102-year-old woman recovered from the infection as well. The majority of people who fall ill will survive.

March 28, 2020

Just 2 weeks ago, we were dealing with 2000 cases of COVID-19 infection and now we have over 100,000. The death toll in Italy has now passed China's reported death toll. In the US, over 2000 people have died with Coronavirus infection, which means that the US death toll has doubled in 2 days. In Chicago, Illinois, an infant who tested positive for COVID-19 has died today. Although a majority of hospitalized patients are adults, we know that children can also be affected. The entire population is at risk. It will not surprise me if we reach a half a million cases in the next 2 weeks. Exponential growth will most certainly test our healthcare system and in some cities, the hospitals will be overwhelmed.

Because so many people are sick, hospitals are using supplies faster than they anticipated. The Coronavirus epidemic did not stop people from getting sick from COPD, pancreatitis, and cancer. There are other medical conditions requiring the same types of supplies and we cannot steal from one group to provide for the other. In some cases, like cleaning supplies, we can substitute needed items with acceptable alternatives. Lysol is literally liquid gold these days as supplies are dwindling. To conserve supply, we are using the CDC-recommended diluted bleach sprays to disinfect rooms between patients. For some supplies such as ventilators, we simply need more. We can move ventilators out of dental surgery offices and outpatient surgery centers into the hospital to increase supply, but in some cities that will not be enough. If you find yourself struggling to breathe and you drive to hospital, you need the ventilator to be at the hospital before you stop breathing … or you die. If the government waits for the illness to surge before ordering the manufacture of needed equipment, people may die while waiting.

The FDA has approved a 15-minute Coronavirus test. Although this is great news, we cannot rest easy after such a small triumph. Imagine what could be accomplished with an ample supply of this test. Instead of banning travel, we can test all incoming passengers and identify those with infection. Instead of banning visitors to nursing homes, we can test all visitors and only turn away the infected. Instead of waiting for hours in a car line for a Coronavirus test, and then wait 4-6 days for results, a person could go to their local clinic and have a visit and results in half an hour. The patients seeking care as well as the staff working aboard the USNS Comfort and USNS Mercy could all be tested to ensure that they aren't going to replicate the disastrous situations of the Princess cruise ships. Having a rapid test is nice but having a rapid test that is widely available is a game-changer.

March 29, 2020

By now you may have realized that social distancing is a method of slowing down the spread of this epidemic. The quarantine is not a cure, so what is being done to actually end this epidemic? Antivirals, antibiotics, passive antibody therapy, and other hospital care are all methods of saving lives, but they do not end the chain of people spreading disease to each other. If we do nothing to stop the spread, eventually everyone will contract the virus and develop natural immunity and the virus will no longer have any hosts to infect.

We would like to return to normal life without having nearly every person become infected with Coronavirus. To accomplish this goal, we would need to ensure that only people free from disease are circulating in society. We can't enjoy a meal in a restaurant if we are worried that the server or staff or the person who sat here before me was carrying Coronavirus. We can't send teachers and students back to school without knowing if anyone is already infected. We already know people feel pressure to go to school or work when sick, and without means of testing

If you are trying to plan for the future by following the messages coming from the Federal Government in DC, you may be confused. Are they planning to loosen social distancing guidelines or are they going to quarantine states and put the people in those states on lockdown? Are they limiting travel between states or are they planning for life to return to normal by Easter? The truth is that your local and state government will determine many of the policies that affect you the most.

The crisis has not yet overwhelmed our city. My coworkers and I are using this time to prepare for the worst. Every hospital, freestanding emergency room, and urgent care clinic has designated rooms and segregated space for treating possible Coronavirus patients to separate them from the general population of patients. My colleagues have researched the different methods of sterilizing used facemasks, just in case we do run out. Apparently, using wet methods of disinfection will degrade the integrity of the fibers and reduce the filtering function of the masks. The preferred methods are using dry heat above 150 degrees Fahrenheit, like from an oven, or hot water vapor from boiling water. Home oven use is not advised, as you would not want to contaminate your home oven with Coronavirus by mistake.

March 30, 2020

This feels like the calm before the storm. The panic in the air has settled. There are no more lines to get into the grocery store. The toilet paper is stacked high on shelves. So are the milk and eggs. Things feel eerily normal … but you can still tell the difference. Today is the first day of online school. After three weeks straight of having all the kids at home, I can't tell if online school is going to make things easier or harder. Can Kindergarten even be successful online? I can't help but feel like the social and emotional development that flourishes in our schools will not transitions well on Zoom video chats.

MYTH: The better we adhere to social distancing, the faster we eradicate Coronavirus.

Social distancing guidelines have been extended nationally through the end of April. I think that people are able to deal with the bad news in small increments. I'm not sure how the country would have handled being told up front that they may have to stay at home for 2-4 months. I definitely think the economy would have reacted poorly to those orders. Still, I see patients who believe that after 2 or 4 or 6 weeks of social distancing, the virus will disappear, and life will return to normal. Unfortunately, the opposite is true. Social distancing slows down the spread and extends the life of the epidemic over a longer time period. Worldwide there are more than 750,000 cases of Coronavirus infection and over 150,000 cases in the United States. There are so many people infected, that it will be nearly impossible for the virus to be eradicated this year. There will always be parts of society that must continue to interact closely with others, and thus, the virus will seek to hang on to that foothold.

I'm hearing that employees for different companies want their jobs closed because a person tests positive for Coronavirus or the employees are threatening to walk out unless they get the hazard pay they want because of the increased danger due to Coronavirus. I wish one of my employees would ask for hazard pay. I always thought hazard pay was for jobs that are more dangerous than the rest, like offshore oilrig workers or contractors who work near a war zone. With Coronavirus, simply being alive is the hazard. Every job has increased risk now. Sitting in a restaurant is potentially hazardous to your health. So is going to church or the gym or to school. Teachers and school nurses wouldn't strike over hazard pay. No one would ask for a grocery store to stay closed indefinitely if an employee tested positive for COVID-19. To some, it may seem reasonable to demand hazard pay when the working conditions increase the risk of illness or death. To others, it is debatable if the workplace is the source of the increased risk, or if the current environment has caused increased risk in every workplace. With unemployment on the rise, I'm shocked people aren't happy to simply have a paying job. I bet there's someone who was recently laid off who's more than willing to do your job without hazard pay.

March 31, 2020

The city and the county continue to open up free testing sites, which is good for everyone. The more people with minimal symptoms who are identified early and kept from spreading to others, the better for all of us. I read that someone proposed we could better isolate the infected by placing them in hotel rooms paid for by the government. I think this would be great for reducing spread of individuals to their families because every family does not have a spare bedroom or garage or basement where a sick family member can isolate away from the rest of the family.

Social distancing is working. Shutting down schools, sporting events, social outings, and restaurants has brought a quick end to this year's flu season as well as the usual spread of other easily transmitted diseases. I haven't seen a positive flu swab test in over a month. In the ER and in Urgent Care, we are seeing fewer and fewer patients. Only the truly sick are coming in for care. This trend is visible all over the country, and local Emergency Rooms and Urgent Care Clinics are either reducing their hours or closing their doors, unable to stay open with such low numbers of patients. Doctors, nurses, and other health professionals are also being laid off or having work hours reduced if they happen to work in areas not directly treating Coronavirus patients.

The US now has suffered more loss of life than China or any other country in the world. Locally, more and more friends and extended family are sharing their experiences with Coronavirus illness and exposure. My coworker who was tested 10 days ago after exposure to a patient who later tested positive, just found out that his test was negative. Can you believe it? An ER doctor on the front lines of the fight against Coronavirus in the 4th largest city in the US had to wait ten days to find out if he has been infected. No matter how far we have come along with improving our testing infrastructure, we still have a long way to go. It makes me think about all of the cities and states reporting low numbers of cases and feeling confident about their situation. If their labs are even 5 days behind, or they don't have an adequate number of tests to administer, they can't possibly even measure the prevalence of infection. They could be sitting in the middle of a local epidemic and not know it.

There is no evidence that any over the counter medication like Advil, Motrin, Ibuprofen, Tylenol, or Acetaminophen cause worse outcomes in patients with Coronavirus. Although the Health Minister of France advised the French people to avoid using anti-inflammatory medicines such as Advil or Motrin the risks of complications are not certain. Severe cases of Coronavirus infection could indirectly lead to kidney damage and high dose use of non-steroid anti-inflammatory medicines could also cause kidney damage.

MYTH: I should avoid Ibuprofen and other anti-inflammatory medications because taking them can make my infection with Coronavirus even worse.

In most cases, patients who are critically ill are not taking over-the-counter medication at the same time. If you have kidney damage, you should be avoiding these medicines already. Most people with Coronavirus infection will not develop kidney failure and do not need to avoid Ibuprofen and other similar medicines.

Another cruise ship is struggling with an outbreak of Coronavirus. The Zandaam is sailing in the Caribbean near

Florida with dozens of symptomatic patients and a handful of confirmed cases of COVID-19. Interesting that the cruise either set sail with Coronavirus test kits or obtained them along the way. Either way, someone was thinking about the spread of Coronavirus, but now the state of Florida is blocking the ship from entering port. We've seen this story before ... the longer the passengers stay aboard, the more people will get the infection, which is bad situation for everyone.

April 1, 2020

Another 30 days of social distancing begins. My neighbors ask me what I think about how and when this all ends. In 30 days, Coronavirus will still be circulating in the population. We may have new treatments by then, like new antiviral medication or convalescent serum or antibody transfer. We may even have enough personal protective equipment (PPE) and ventilators to properly supply our hospital workers and first responders. Even with all of these assumptions, we will not have any new method of keeping the virus from spreading from one person to another. In 30 days, we may see the number of cases rise and plateau, and some people will feel better and say that the worst is behind us. No matter what people say, you should know this – we are using social distancing because distance is the best tool, next to hand hygiene, that we have to reduce the spread of this disease. Once the protective distancing recommendations are removed, the virus will spread again. If we do not have adequate tests to identify the asymptomatic carriers of the virus, we are likely to see an unexpected increase in cases of infection.

My wife's best friend just found out her mother has COVID-19. For over a week, she has been concerned about her mother not eating, feeling weak and tired, having intermittent fevers, and complaining of aches and pains for almost 2 weeks now. She has no history of travel outside of the city of Houston and had adhered to the stay at home guidelines from the day they were announced. Over a week ago, she was tested for COVID-19 and they found out today that she is positive. Even though we do not have a prescription to help treat it, there is peace of mind that comes with knowing the cause of your loved one's suffering.

My neighbor who works for a car dealership told me an interesting story today. A couple from Washington, not far from Seattle, travelled all the way here to buy a pre-owned E550 Sedan. They wore masks and gloves, confirmed the car looked as advertised before buying it, then drove back home to Washington. This is how seriously they wanted a car with less risk of Coronavirus. People are getting the message. Social distancing is the new way of life.

April 2, 2020

All my kids are staying up past midnight and waking up later and later. The website that is supposed to host the educational interaction between my kids and their teachers doesn't work in the mornings, probably because there are

100,000 other parents trying to use it at the same time. Meanwhile, over a million people around the world have tested positive for COVID-19, and probably a million more people who had it and were never tested. The national testing companies are reporting a backlog of over 100,000 test kits waiting to be processed. A thousand people or more a day are dying from this disease, and we barely have any tools to stop it. The worst part is that the better we distance ourselves socially and stay at home, the longer we suffer this upswing of sickness. Still, a slow climb is the better option, as a fast rise in illness will overwhelm our hospitals.

We have not run out of ventilators in the US. This means that most likely the people who have died were already on a ventilator. People are starting to wonder how a patient can die while on a ventilator. A ventilator is a device that supplies oxygenated air with significant positive pressure to inflate the lungs. This allows better oxygen delivery to the lung tissue in an attempt to improve the amount of oxygen circulating in our blood. However, it does not improve the heart's ability to pump and circulate blood or the kidneys' ability to filter and clean the blood. Other organ systems can fail while the body suffers a severe infection. A ventilator can help someone survive a critical illness, but a ventilator is not the cure for this disease.

My coworker hasn't seen her son in 2 weeks. She is an ER nurse and ICU nurse and her ex-husband doesn't want their kid exposed to Coronavirus. Our front-line defenders around the country are isolating themselves from family and friends to reduce risk of community spread and we must applaud them for this. But we must also face reality. How long can a person suffer being isolated from family and friends? How long can society survive sheltering in place? Whether we shutter society for a month or a season or the rest of the year, Coronavirus will be here. We were never ahead of this virus. We only found patients after they got sick. We still can't see the people who are carrying it with mild or no symptoms. When we do return to life as we knew it, the virus will still be hiding in plain sight.

April 3, 2020

The Governor of Texas has extended the statewide closure of schools until the first week of May, but we already knew that was coming. My oldest son really misses school, which totally took me by surprise. The Governor of Georgia has issued statewide stay at home orders, one of the last in the country to do so, after proclaiming that he just recently learned about asymptomatic spreading of Coronavirus. An ostrich with his head in the sand cannot see a nearby threat until it's too late. We have known about people spreading Coronavirus without symptoms for months now, which is why there are so many sick people in so many places. In fact, if your town, city, or state does not have an outbreak of Coronavirus, you probably don't have adequate testing where you are. In Ecuador, bodies are literally piling up in the streets. Today, Houston opens its second public testing site for Coronavirus for any and all residents. Every leader who isn't in the middle of an epidemic right now must decide if the lessons from Italy, New York, and Ecuador will guide them to test early and identify the problem, or if the virus will rise up first and show us the problem cannot be contained.

In the last 2 weeks, over 10 million Americans have lost their jobs, and many have also lost their health insurance. Roughly half of American adults have some kind of pre-existing medical condition. The wheels are in motion and we may be heading toward a different kind of health crisis. How will people keep their diabetes and high blood pressure and asthma under control if they don't have insurance to help cover costs of medications and doctor visits? How will people afford replacement insurance plans if the Affordable Care Act marketplaces are not an option? The time to address these questions is now, while people still have their current medications.

Fortunately, Congress has passed the largest bill in history, now signed into law by the President, to provide much needed financial relief to struggling people and struggling businesses alike. Healthcare in this country is still fundamentally linked to employment for more than half of Americans. High rates of unemployment lead to higher rates of people being uninsured, which could be life-threatening in this time of this global health emergency. The financial support provided to small businesses and large corporations hopefully keep people employed during these tough times. The mandated increase in unemployment payments will help keep people in their homes with bills paid and refrigerators replenished. The stimulus check payments should provide a financial boost for a sluggish economy and help ensure the underemployed still have money for their household necessities. So many people suffer from medical conditions like high blood pressure and diabetes, it's easy to see that a lapse in steady income would put their health in jeopardy.

The US Government Coronavirus Task Force is reporting that Coronavirus particles can be transmitted person to person through the act of speaking, not just coughing or sneezing. We all know someone who spits a bit when they talk. Hopefully, those are the only ones spreading disease with speaking. The US already has over 250,000 confirmed cases and an unknown number of mild or asymptomatic cases. If viral shedding is occurring with normal speech and breathing, then we are in for a tough road ahead.

It seems like social distancing is transforming into a Shutdown Syndrome. I agree with the current closings of schools and businesses, but I hear some suggesting that essential services close because an employee tests positive for COVID-19. Are we really releasing inmates and prisoners because a guard or an inmate tests positive for Coronavirus? What if the police department or fire department closed because a person tested positive? When schools return to normal business, will we close them when a teacher or student tests positive? At some point, we must proceed through different stages of adjustment and arrive at acceptance. We cannot eradicate this virus, no matter how hard we try, and so we must learn to live with it.

The FDA has given emergency authorization for use of a new COVID-19 test that would identify the presence of IgG and IgM antibodies to COVID-19. The test uses a small blood sample, similar to a blood sugar test, and measures the presence or absence of these antibodies in only 15 minutes. The previous test using nasal swabs looked for active infection. This new test for antibodies can also identify immunity. After a person passes beyond the asymptomatic stage of infection and enters symptomatic disease, the IgM antibody is produced. As the illness resolves and the person begins to recover, the IgM starts to fade away while the body begins to produce the antibody IgG. Even after full recovery, IgG levels persist and provide protection against future infection. Although we do not know how many weeks or months the IgG for Coronavirus will last, because this is a new infection for everyone, we can safely assume that the presence of both IgM and IgG indicate active infection and IgG alone indicates declining or past infection. If no antibodies are present, either there has been no infection or very early infection is present. A rapid antibody test will be essential in our goal of returning to a sense of normalcy, because people with immunity will feel reassured in returning to the workforce.

April 4, 2020

Decades ago, the world did not have a safe and widely available vaccine for Chickenpox. When you talk to older Americans, most of them suffered from the virus at some point in their childhood. This is part of the reason why so many older adults suffer from Shingles, a reactivation of the Chickenpox virus. Once the vaccine was created and approved in the US in the 1990s, the younger generations were protected from Chickenpox. Similarly, since we do not have a vaccine for Coronavirus, we should expect everyone to become infected. It's only a matter of time. It is uncertain if an unlimited supply of masks and ventilators or an unlimited amount of chloroquine and azithromycin will prevent everyone from getting the infection. With any luck, an effective vaccine can be created by next year, but until then, we are faced with two options – do everything we can to slow the spread until the vaccine is ready or return to some form of normal societal interaction and accept the consequences. Both scenarios are dreadful for our society and our economy.

MYTH: We are just now learning that Coronavirus can spread from infected people who do not have symptoms.

Universal mask usage is now advised as an optional method of slowing the spread of Coronavirus. Although people are saying that we are just now learning that people can spread the infection with no symptoms or minimal symptoms, we first suspected asymptomatic spread in

January when people in California became infected despite having no travel history. As more and more people appeared around the country with Coronavirus infection without history of recent travel, suspicion of asymptomatic spread grew. In cities where populations are dense or cities with large public gatherings, we have seen exponential rise of cases of infection. We do not have data yet on how many viral particles are spread when these symptomless spreaders talk or breathe, but we can assume that people are spreading infection before displaying symptoms based on how rapidly the virus is spreading despite the great efforts taken to attempt to identify all contacts of an infected individual.

The US now has over 300,000 cases of infection and over 8000 deaths from COVID-19, we also see that 49 of our 50 states have lost lives from the infection. Over 1.2 million people have Coronavirus infection, with no signs of worldwide spread slowing down. All eyes are focused on the place we believe the infection started as we watch to see how the lockdown measures are lifted. While other parts of China have somewhat returned to normal, the people in Wuhan, China are still waiting for lockdown to be lifted. Their residents will eventually be allowed to return to some form of normalcy, but the world will be watching to see if new cases of Coronavirus infection emerge. The best way for the US to plan a method of easing social distancing would be monitor the actions taken by other countries to learn what steps are effective and what measures cause setbacks.

The White House Coronavirus Task Force has informed us that for the safety of the President, all members of the Task Force are getting the COVID-19 rapid test on a daily basis. In doing so, they have silently revealed a bitter truth that they have not formally announced ... to return to business as usual, to have usual working relationships, to function normally and not put the life of the President at risk, all of the people who come in contact with the President must be tested on a regular basis. Let's apply this fact to everyone else in America. If we want to return to life as normal, we would need to test people for the disease on an ongoing basis, not just once or twice, which means we would need to run hundreds of millions of tests every day and get same-day results. The truth is that America needs a billion tests by the end of the year, and we are nowhere near that reality today.

April 5, 2020

Today is Palm Sunday. We did church by video streaming today. Church services virtually is the only safe way to go during this pandemic. The risk of attending a large group function is too great. Fortunately, most people are taking this seriously and exhibiting self-discipline with social distancing. GPS data from Google shows that in majority of states, people are moving around much less than usual. Unfortunately, some people do not have the option of practicing social distancing as well as other. Every nursing home is filled with people who rely on the close contact of others on a daily basis. The residents of some nursing homes rarely leave the home. In the previous nursing home outbreaks, most people concluded that the staff must have brought the virus into the nursing home and spread to the residents. In every case that has been reported, once the Coronavirus was introduced into the nursing home, over half of residents contracted the virus within a month. Many of those infected residents have required hospitalization for care. Unless we test every person who goes into a nursing home every day, it is only a matter of time before every nursing home suffers the same fate. The same situation will likely occur in jails and prisons, where people are unable to comply with social distancing.

A scientific study from 2010 conducted by the US and the Netherlands reported that researchers used Zinc ions in combination with pyrithione, a zinc ionophore, given in low concentration to inhibit the replication of SARS-Coronavirus in cultured cells infected with SARS-Coronavirus. They used a Zinc solution with 500 micromolar (micromoles per liter) concentration and pyrithione to act as a transport mechanism to allow the zinc to pass through the viral cell wall. Imagine a crowded event with long lines and heavy security. The pyrithione acts like a VIP pass that allows the guest, zinc, to enter the venue much more quickly. Without pyrithione, the zinc molecule would have difficulty passing through the virus cell wall. Interestingly enough, Chloroquine is also a zinc ionophore, which means that it also would allow zinc to enter the viral cell in higher amounts than usual. Given the molecular weight of Zinc is 65.38 grams and the typical volume of serum in an adult is 5 or 6 L, in theory it would take a daily dose of about 200mg of elemental Zinc to raise normal serum concentration of a person to the target concentration of 500 micromoles per liter. The hope would be that the same approach would inhibit replication of COVID-19.

Unfortunately, the human body is more complex than the controlled environment of cultured cells in a laboratory. Over 99% of the zinc in a person's body is stored in the skeletal system. Ingestion of zinc in doses greater than 10 milligrams leads to increased excretion of the zinc more than increased absorption. The majority of zinc intake is either taken into the bone for storage or dumped out of the body through the intestinal system. Only a small fraction remains in the serum, and this complex system would make it nearly impossible to achieve the optimal serum zinc concentration to effectively inhibit replication of Coronavirus. Furthermore, prolonged use of elevated doses of zinc have been shown to cause copper deficiency, anemia, and even impaired immune function. The studies did show that the lower concentrations of zinc treatments were less effective, not ineffective. Concentrations of 100 micromoles per liter were substantially effective and could be achieved in bursts by taking 40 mg of elemental zinc once or twice a day. Zinc sulfate and zinc acetate are preferred over zinc oxide and zinc carbonate, which do not dissolve and absorb as easily. Be sure to check the back label of your supplement bottle.

In Italy, doctors have been reporting that patients who received hydroxychloroquine and azithromycin have made miraculous recoveries after severe illness with COVID-19. In a clinical study in China, published in February of 2020, doctors randomly assigned COVID-19 patients to receive standard treatment with antibiotics, antivirals, immune globulin, and supportive care or receive standard treatment plus hydroxychloroquine (HCQ) 200mg twice a day for 5 days. The patients who received standard care plus HCQ demonstrated shorter times to clinical recovery and were more likely to have pneumonia resolve in shorter timeframe. The CDC is currently authorizing the use of chloroquine (CQ), hydroxychloroquine, azithromycin (Zpak) and other drugs for use in hospitalized patients and for use in clinical trials designed to study the effectiveness of treatment of COVID-19. If any of these combinations of zinc and chloroquine or hydroxychloroquine and azithromycin are effective at treating early disease, we would need to manufacture these medicines locally and in high quantities. If they can be proven effective at prevention, the need for an ample supply of the medication would grow even more.

April 6, 2020

As the country heads toward 350,000 cases of COVID-19 infections and 10,000 COVID-19 related deaths, we are bracing for the "worst week ever" dealing with this infection. Despite last week being the worst week we had seen thus far, this week will probably be worse, and the following week after may be worse still. We are still slowly moving up the first hill of this rollercoaster, the big hill, and just like on a roller coaster, you may not be able to see the top. It's not until you reach the apex and head down that you realize you were just at the peak. We may or may not feel a change when we reach the top, but one day, we will be able to look back and see that the worst is behind us. Will there be more peaks? It is probable, especially when children return to school and large social gatherings resume. After the virus was under control in South Korea and China, social restrictions were loosened and subsequently, they saw rises in new cases of infection. New York may reach a peak in cases this week, but most of the country will not. In Houston, we are just at the beginning of the rise of infection. Right now is the best time to plan and prepare for life after the peak.

To prevent a second rise in cases after relaxing social distancing recommendations, we may have to rely on universal mask usage to reduce the spread from asymptomatic cases and protect the general public. In addition, we will need adequate testing to identify the ill quickly. In a country of over 320 million people, we will need hundreds of millions of tests. By providing effective treatment for patients early in the course of the disease, we can reduce the severity of each illness and reduce the number of days of viral shedding, thereby decreasing the potential spread of infection. Wearing a mask does not replace social distancing, rather, it adds to it's effectiveness. By combining all these efforts, we may have an effective approach to controlling the spread of Coronavirus while allowing life to return to some version of normal.

Although Chloroquine (CQ) and Hydroxychloroquine (HCQ) are being studied as treatment for COVID-19, it is not likely that this could be used as a daily preventive method. Currently, CQ and HCQ are FDA approved for prevention and treatment of malaria. The prevention dosing schedule advises one pill a week for two weeks prior to a trip to any place where malaria is common. Now that Coronavirus is actively spreading in the community of nearly every major city, a person would need to take any preventive measures from now until the threat passed. Prevention works best when an undesirable disease can be prevented with a low dose of a relatively nontoxic medication. For chronic recurrent urinary tract infections, a low dose of an antibiotic has been used as a daily prophylactic. A low dose of an antiviral is also currently used as a daily prophylactic for herpetic cold sores. In both of these cases, a patient must use it for the rest of his or her lifetime.

MYTH: I can take Chloroquine or Hydroxychloroquine daily to protect myself from getting COVID-19.

Thousands of people are already using these medicines on a daily basis for treatment of lupus and other arthritis. It is possible to study these individuals to find out if they develop typical symptoms of COVID-19 infection, a milder case, or no infection at all. I have taken both CQ and HCQ in the past, once for treatment of malaria as a teen, and once for prevention several years ago. I speak from experience when I say that the side effects are not pleasant. Common side effects include nausea, vomiting, and crampy abdominal pain. Rare side effects include vertigo, tinnitus, and muscle weakness. Prolonged use of the medications can lead to progressive and irreversible eye disease that may progress to blindness. A medication with high potential for side effects and significant risk of irreversible damage with prolonged use is unlikely to be approved for daily preventive treatment. More scientific studies are needed to determine proper dosing for CQ and HCQ of if they are even reliably effective at treating COVID-19. Without this additional validation, no one will be discussing these two drugs as a serious option for prevention.

Another week of online school from home. I just don't feel like this is optimal learning for Kindergarten. 6-year-olds can't use Zoom for web conferencing by themselves and they can't log into Schoology by themselves either. They enjoy seeing each other on the computer, but a few hours a week of group facetime is nothing compared to the 30 hours of fundamental teaching and social interaction they would normally be getting. As much as I fear the return of school for the spread of the virus that will follow, I can't wait for school to be back in session.

April 7, 2020

Telemedicine is all the rage right now. As the number of Coronavirus infections approaches 400,000, people are avoiding emergency room and clinics as much as possible. A mother contacted our clinic with concerns for her son's painful and swollen testicle. In normal times, people would rush into the ER or the nearest clinic for a prompt evaluation for this type of problem. Through the video chat, I could see that one side of the scrotum was swollen and red and the child's face indicated significant pain. I had no choice but to advise a prompt trip to the ER for ultrasound. Upon follow up, we learned that the testicle had to be removed due to inadequate blood flow for too long. The pain had started the night before, but everyone is hesitant to go to the hospital these days. The Coronavirus pandemic is affecting our lives in ways we could not have predicted.

UK Prime Minister Boris Johnson has reportedly been moved to the ICU for treatment of his COVID-19 infection. I imagine that every investigational drug and every proposed but untested treatment combo is being considered. They will want to do everything possible to ensure his speedy recovery. Surprisingly, the UK spokesperson for the Prime Minister reports that Mr. Johnson is breathing without mechanical assistance, meaning no ventilator is being used, and that he does not have pneumonia. This is good news as many of the COVID-19 patients in ICUs around the country are on ventilators and many have pneumonia. Hopefully, he recovers quickly without needing any additional critical care.

Over 1800 Americans lost their lives today to Coronavirus, the most so far in this country's pandemic. New York also reported their highest one-day death toll yesterday. We are all hopeful for the peak of this journey, but these new figures are sobering. We have evidence that social distancing is working in several cities where the number of cases continues to rise very slowly. The number of new cases of COVID-19 infection in New York has remained relatively the same over the past few days. Smaller hotspots around the country are also reporting a similar trend. In contrast, there are other cities with rapidly rising infection where the virus is setting the timetable and contradicting the shifting forecasts from the experts.

April 8, 2020

People are asking me why the prediction models for Coronavirus keep changing. Forecasting the future is a difficult task. In terms of hurricanes, we have decades of data on previous hurricanes that help shape those predictions. We do not have the same level of data on viruses like COVID-19 that spread across the globe in months. It would be very valuable to have an accurate forecast on the number of sick patients each week to help plan and prepare an adequate amount of supplies and hospital beds. Unfortunately, prediction models for this new virus will likely all be wrong, but some will be less wrong than others.

Accurately predicting the future is nearly impossible, but properly interpreting current data can also be difficult. For example, in New York, they reported a rise in the number of deaths yesterday, a rise in the number of new cases, and a fall in the number of hospitalized COVID-19 patients on a ventilator. A reduction in the number of people in critical care units using a ventilator seems like good news at first glance. If the reduction occurs completely because patients are recovering from the disease, that would be the best possible outcome. However, when a patient worsens and passes away, that also reduces the count of patients with COVID-19 using a ventilator. More unused ventilators do not always mean something good is happening. Without knowing the details behind the numbers, one cannot assume that the changes indicate good or bad things.

MYTH: Screening the general public by measuring temperatures will identify all possible Coronavirus carriers.

Several airlines and workplaces are screening people by questionnaire and measuring their clients' temperatures prior to entry. This is not a bad idea, but it is also not an effective method of screening out people who have Coronavirus. Every ER physician I know has seen a patient who did not have fever and ended up testing positive for Coronavirus. Patients with COVID-19 are telling their own stories on social media and many reveal that they tested positive for a second time after a 14-day quarantine. So few people are receiving follow up testing after infection, it is not clear what percentage of infections will last longer than 14 days.

April 9, 2019

All of the places I work will be getting access to a limited amount of Coronavirus testing. This indicates a remarkable improvement in testing supply, but it also gives hope that we are finally attempting to catch up to the demand for testing. Anyone who believes we have been testing adequately in this country is sadly mistaken. At one job, a rapid test for active COVID-19 disease will be used to help differentiate the admitted patients whose symptoms make it unclear if they have Coronavirus or not. By reducing the number of patients requiring isolation and Coronavirus-related protection measures, we reduce the use of the valuable protective equipment that all healthcare providers will need. At another facility, the tests are used based on the decision-making of the provider and the clinical presentation of the patient, which gives people an opportunity to advocate for themselves in hopes of finding out if they are infected or not. In another facility, the tests are administered in conjunction with the local health department to provide testing to individuals with symptoms or persons with high risk of complications from Coronavirus infection. Each place has a different directive guiding the testing administration, and that underscores the fact that no one has enough tests to simply test everyone who's a reasonable suspect for COVID-19 infection.

MYTH: If I test negative for Coronavirus, I'm clear from disease and I don't have to worry about being infected.

No test is perfect. All testing is flawed in some way. A clinician must learn the flaws of a test in order to use the test properly. Many people know that a pregnancy test could be falsely negative if it is performed too early in the pregnancy. The same phenomenon occurs with flu testing and most likely applies to Coronavirus testing as well. But a pregnancy test can also be falsely positive. Some tumors secrete hormones of pregnancy and can cause a false-positive pregnancy test. Luckily, we can use an ultrasound to confirm pregnancy and guard against false positive tests. For Coronavirus, we would have to use a second test to confirm results if we were concerned about false results. Unfortunately, we do not have enough tests for people to have a second test routinely. This is also why we are unable to routinely test for cure after patients have recovered after an infection with COVID-19. Patients who test negative at one point in time may be exposed to the virus in the future and contract the disease. It is also possible to test negative for disease but have the virus in your system at an early stage of infection. A negative test provides information about the past, not necessarily about the present, and definitely not about the future.

In the coming weeks, cities around the country will see the number of Coronavirus cases flatten and in some cities they will fall. When that happens, the leaders of those cities and states will have a choice to make. Will they proclaim that social distancing is working and double-down and continue the measures or will they proclaim victory over Coronavirus and relax the social distancing measures? In Spain and Italy, where they hope to reach a peak in cases of infection soon, we will be watching to see how they respond to the same question. The government of China has relaxed restrictions on the people of Wuhan, the city that suffered the first epidemic of COVID-19. They are reportedly using a complex smartphone app with GPS location tracking to monitor each person's activity with the ability to inform individuals in real time about their risk of being infected based on proximity to others who have recently tested positive.

In the US, we do not yet have any similar method of population tracking and no way to do rapid contact tracing. Over 450,000 people have confirmed infection with COVID-19. Even if we imagine there are 4 or 5 more people with unconfirmed infection for every confirmed case, that only takes us to about 3 million cases of infection. That still leaves over 320 million potential targets for the virus without a vaccine to protect them. In cities with regular use of public transportation or high frequency of large gatherings, we may see infection spread again.

April 10, 2020

Some would say that looking backwards during these times of crisis is not effective use of time. However, those who do not learn from history are doomed to repeat it. Researchers have been reviewing the genetic code of COVID-19 from different patients in New York and they have identified spelling errors that occur when the virus replicate. By comparing these spelling errors to other outbreak clusters, they have deduced that the epidemic in New York likely originated from over half-a-dozen different initial patients who likely traveled in from Europe in late January. This is more evidence that the virus has been circulating right before our eyes while inadequate testing blinds us from seeing a clear picture of the disease.

There are some people who believe we will not need widespread testing to return to a normal level of daily interaction. This may be true currently, but we must also look ahead. Most people are anticipating a normal school year in the fall. We would also anticipate a typical flu season starting in the late fall. If we do not have easy access to same day test results for Coronavirus testing, how will we handle sick patients during next cold and flu season? Will every child with a cough need to stay home for 14 days? Will every teacher do the same? Will nursing home employees test for Coronavirus or only check their temperatures? The second wave of infections that we will likely see this summer will be different from the third wave of infections we see during the late fall and early winter.

Clinics were already seeing employees sent home for coughing or sneezing and advised to return only when cleared by a physician even before immunity testing had been developed. Employers are not willing to risk the health and safety of their workforce on the chance that a person with dry cough and runny nose has seasonal allergies and not COVID-19. With adequate supply, it's possible that large employers may self-fund the testing of their employees. As a country with nearly half a million cases of Coronavirus infection and over 18,000 deaths from the virus, we have already seen what happens when the population behaves normally without knowing who is carrying the disease. Going forward, we must plan appropriately for the return of normalcy or we will fall victim to the return of Coronavirus.

For days the media has been reporting on mortality statistics released by several cities and counties in hotspots around the country. These statistics indicate that the percentage of African American deaths due to COVID-19 out of total deaths due to COVID-19 is several times greater than the percentage of African Americans in the population in these same areas. In cities where African Americans are less than 25% of the population, they may be 50% or more of the deaths associated with COVID-19. This would not be the first time that a disease affects a subset of a population more than others, but we cannot easily explain differences in survival rate with differences in race. Diabetes, heart disease, and some forms of cancer all affect minorities at higher rates than the general public, but they also affect people of lower socio-economic status more than others.

MYTH: The Coronavirus affects all racial, social, and economic groups equally.

Earning a lower income may inhibit a person's ability to maintain social distancing. A person who has to ride a train or a bus to get to work has less ability to socially distance compared to people who drive or people who are able to work from home. People who are able to have groceries delivered can avoid the risk of close contact with strangers at the supermarket. Access to healthcare is another important factor that may increase the risk of some people over others. Due to the backlog of send-out nasal swab tests, patients already in the hospital have been getting COVID-19 test results days earlier than people who went to county drive-up testing centers. A patient recently told me that she visited the local country drive-up testing location for three days straight, arriving at 5:00 AM on the third day in order to get a good place in line to be able to get tested. Luckily, she tested negative and she remained healthy. A delay of several days with inadequate supportive care could be the difference between getting on the road to recovery or going into the ICU for critical care. Dissecting the data on the comorbidities and the demographics of the deceased will shed some light on how to identify high-risk patients so that we could intervene earlier and advise hospitalization instead of home care.

April 11, 2020

Today the country has over 500,000 cases of infection and

only about 2.5 million tests have been performed. Two weeks ago, the country only had 100,000 cases, and despite social distancing in most of the country for a month, the disease continues to spread. As Easter approaches, people are longing for social interaction and longing to get out of the house. The Governor of Texas has given churches the right to hold mass and other religious services, but social distancing recommendations would still classify attending church as a potentially risky activity. Despite the risk, people want to get back to work. The government cannot financially support every family and it cannot educate every child from home indefinitely. I have quietly come to accept the likelihood that in-class school will not be resuming this school year. A return to work necessitates a return of some form of routine school and childcare, which means that the decision to reduce or end social distancing will be made by groups of leaders at both regional and local levels.

A recent abstract published in the New England Journal of Medicine on the effects of Remdesivir offered some much-needed hope in the midst of these trying times. Remdesivir is a new antiviral drug that is being studied in several institutions around the world for its potential effectiveness in treating patients with COVID-19. In this study, a 10-day course the drug was delivered intravenously to 53 patients with confirmed COVID-19 disease with documented low oxygen saturation levels or need for supplemental oxygen. Standard treatment for respiratory infections was also provided to all patients. After two to three weeks of follow-up, over two-thirds of these patients showed clinical improvement in the amount of oxygen-support they needed. Over half of the patients on ventilator support were breathing without the ventilator during the same follow-up period. Although researchers must study the effects of this drug in a randomized controlled trial to prove a significant benefit, we are all happy to see more new drugs with the possibility of helping COVID-19 patients recover more quickly.

Looking forward into the summer and fall, how will any organization host a large gathering safely? Can a sporting event or a concert screen thousands of guests in a few hours? The country doesn't have enough tests for current needs, so testing people at social events seems improbable. Measuring temperature on entry may screen out some ill guests, but patients carrying COVID-19 with no symptoms will slip past this line of defense and still potentially expose everyone sitting nearby. Even if we move to universal mask usage, I don't know how well that would work with cheering fans consuming food and beverages and celebrating together. Sports teams may be playing in stadiums full of people wearing mask or stadiums full of empty seats, depending on our ability to test and treat this disease.

April 13, 2020

The outbreak in New York continues to make up nearly half of the cases of infection and nearly half of the deaths for the whole country, yet New York has only 6% of the country's population. Will the epidemic in New York be the example that every major city follows or is it somehow a one-time event? To put things in a proper perspective, despite everything we have endured thus far, less than 1% of the nation's population has tested positive for this virus. Social distancing has slowed the spread of the infection to allow hospitals to prepare and for scientists to develop new technologies to test and devise new ways of treating COVID-19. Is it possible that the country has seen the worst of this virus when so many people are still vulnerable? Even if we assume that the virus is present in 10% of the population, that leaves 90% of the nation at risk, with no vaccine or other antibody treatment to provide protection from infection.

Brazilian scientists recently posted results from a research study in which 81 patients presumed to have COVID-19 were randomized into a high-dose chloroquine treatment group or a low-dose chloroquine treatment group. Every patient in the study also received azithromycin and ceftriaxone, antibiotics commonly used in treatment of pneumonia. All of the patients were hospitalized adults with one or more of the following: rapid heart rate, rapid breathing, low oxygen saturation, or shock. Only some of the patients were confirmed COVID-19 positive before inclusion into the study. Physicians and patients were not aware of the group assignment of any patient; medications were prepared by the pharmacy with placebo pills used as needed. Three days into the study, several patients developed abnormal heart rhythms. The study was halted prematurely after nearly a dozen patients died, and they found that the deaths occurred in the high-dose treatment group.

The results of this study are very different from the earlier studies that showed success with critically ill patients recovering rapidly from COVID-19 infection. However, this study brought to light the risks of chloroquine use and the outcomes suggest that the risk increases with the dose used. The study did not prove effectiveness of the low-dose regimen due to the small size of the study and the abrupt end. The researchers highlighted the proposed mechanisms of action of broad-spectrum antiviral effects of chloroquine directly interfering with the way SARS-Coronavirus binds with human cells. Interestingly, they did not highlight the other mechanism of action that was proven effective against SARS-Coronavirus, where chloroquine allowed zinc ions into the virus cell to halt viral replication. Many believe that CQ and HCQ will directly attack and kill COVID-19 cells, but it is also possible that they simply act as a Trojan Horse that allows zinc into the viral cell interior. Further review of the differences between studies will hopefully lead to better treatment plans in the future. As the US approaches 600,000 cases of infection and 25,000 deaths, and the world approaches 2 million cases of infection, everyone is depending on it.

Dr. Xavier Odili

Coronavirus on my Mind – Part 2

We have known for months that the working class, the women of our country, and the peoples of color in America are at higher risk of contracting COVID-19 for many reasons. The types of jobs that cannot be performed from home, the types of jobs where social distancing is nearly impossible, and the home life situations where an infected person cannot distance from family to protect them all contribute to that increased risk. We also know that the differences in the way some people in these groups access and interact with our healthcare system that led to higher rate of death in minorities from diabetes and heart disease would translate into higher death rate from COVID-19 as well. Despite these facts, we are seeing a crisis of misinformation spreading faster than the virus. Some people don't believe the virus is real. Some people don't think the virus is hurting anyone. Some people think the death toll is exaggerated. The images of large crowds of people at parties and inside bars and clubs are disturbing.

As a healthcare provider, I plead to you today to think twice before you underestimate this virus. If not for yourself, then for your neighbors, your extended family, and your coworkers. You may not die from a COVID-19 infection, in fact, you may not even notice if you are infected, but if you pass the infection to a friend or family member who isn't as lucky, you can't take that back. The truths of COVID-19 must be spread to dispel the rumors and myths in hopes that we continue to slow the spread of infection until a vaccine is developed.

Chapter 6

The USA Collectively Holds its Breath

April 16, 2020

Life seems to have slowed to a crawl. The hustle and bustle of normal life has gone quiet in many places. The economy wasn't turned off like a light switch – this was more like ripping the switch out of the wall. We can't just flip life back to the way it used to be. Getting things back to normal will not be simple. We are all waiting to find out what happens next, and the uncertainty is unsettling. Some of our leaders are going to underestimate the gravity of the situation that faces us in the future. This is why it is so important that our elected officials have great intelligence and great experience. Governing is easier when everything is going well. However, in times of disaster, experience and intelligence will determine if the end result is success or failure.

April 17, 2020

In cities with high numbers of hospitalizations, their public health departments may not have the luxury of testing individuals with little or no symptoms. Testing supplies are a limited resource. Like all limited resources, organizations develop rules to help preserve the resource so that it can be used in the best manner possible and to avoid running out of the resource in time of need. If you become ill, you would like for there to be a test available to you. In large cities, this means that tests are likely not available to people without symptoms. Patients who are concerned about potential exposure are advised to self-quarantine at home for 14 days. With an unlimited testing supply, these patients would be tested before being sent home to quarantine, tested again if they develop symptoms at any time during the 2 weeks, and if still negative, tested at the end of the 14 days. In our current situation, we can only test a person with symptoms. Most patients without symptoms can avoid an empty trip to the hospital for testing which also means avoiding additional exposure to COVID-19.

April 19, 2020

Sadly, the country passed new milestones during the COVID-19 pandemic with 40,000 American deaths and over 750,000 cases of infection. Sad, but not unexpected. Every city is looking for more testing capability, but US manufacturing cannot meet these demands. Many of COVID-19 tests, swabs, and supporting materials are manufactured overseas, but this is not new knowledge. For decades, American manufacturing companies have willingly shifted away from making products in America to cut costs and maximize profits. The factories that once thrived in the Midwest and other parts of the country have been sitting idle for years. The worldwide increase in demand for medical supplies will likely last for years. Our unemployed workforce is looking for work opportunities and our country is desperate for local manufacturing of essential medical equipment for the current pandemic and for our security and preparedness for the pandemics of the future.

The lack of local manufacturing forced the country to rely on foreign-manufactured tests. This vulnerability has already led to negative consequences. In Laredo, Texas, the local government leaders partnered with an emergency room owner to purchase 20,000 COVID-19 tests. Earlier this month, those tests were validated and found to be unreliable, therefore unusable, and then seized by the government. Last week in Memphis, Tennessee, the government seized a shipment of fake COVID-19 tests arriving from China. The FDA released a warning to the general public for anyone attempting to purchase COVID-19 tests to beware of counterfeit tests or home delivery tests. The FDA at this time has not given authorization for any home administered COVID test of any kind, although the idea is being considered.

MYTH: All COVID-19 antibody tests are faulty and prone to give false positive or false negative results.

No test is perfect. It's reasonable to have concern about the accuracy of any test that you take. A pregnancy test will always be validated by an ultrasound later. A screening HIV test will be validated by a second confirmatory test. A mammogram that suggests a tumor will be validated by a biopsy. We already understand that every test has a risk of false results. The real question should be how much is that risk of false results. Only the data can answer that question. Fears are rising among the public after reports of several COVID-19 tests being sold with high rates of test result inaccuracies. I have read about the fears, but I have not seen any data showing high rates of false results. Data is data. However, if someone is concerned, that person can request and read the data behind a test, or at least ask someone who has read the data. Antibody testing is not an emergency need. If someone is afraid, they should not take a test they do not trust. As research continues, testing accuracy will improve, and better tests will hopefully be developed here in the USA.

April 20, 2020

Throughout this pandemic, we have observed other countries of the world to find the best methods for containing this virus. Monitoring the trends of other countries can give insight into our future with COVID-19. Singapore initially contained the spread of COVID-19 using social distancing laws and other isolation techniques. After they relaxed social distancing, the numbers of infected persons have risen and yesterday reported their highest number of new cases ever seen. Specifically, many of the new cases have been found in the essential factory and construction workers and the migrant working class in Singapore. This is not surprising given everything we know and have already seen about Coronavirus. Your ability to maintain a good distance from your coworkers depends heavily on the type of work that you do.

Over the past week, reported deaths due to COVID-19 has doubled from 21000 to 42000. While the disease seems to be spreading less in New York, it is clearly spreading more in other localities. Even if there is not a rapid increase in your local area, the potential for spread remains. In fact, we are likely to see cities yo-yo up and down between phases of controlled disease and uncontrolled spread for many months to come.

April 21, 2020

A ban on immigration has been proposed ... not a ban on international travel ... as if one can determine who might have Coronavirus based on immigration status. I am not sure how blocking immigrants is going to help us acquire the testing kits and supplies that we seem to be unable to manufacture here in the US. To focus your attention on a nonexistent incoming threat also draws your attention away from the threat that has been here for so long.

Contact tracing surveillance will be a key element in the efforts to prevent future outbreaks after social distancing is relaxed. Many countries were able to quickly interview infected patients to identify family, friends, and other people who were exposed to the virus through close proximity or direct contact with the patient. A successful application of this practice was the key to preventing widespread infection in the countries like South Korea and Japan. Months ago, the exposed parties would be placed on a 14-day home quarantine and monitored for symptoms. We now know that not everyone who is exposed to an infected individual will contract the infection. With prompt contact tracing, we may see a combination of rapid testing for disease and for antibodies and a much shorter quarantine with retesting for active disease a week later replace the old method of 2-week isolation.

Contact tracing has limitations. People do not know the names of everyone they pass in the grocery store or the people standing behind them in line for coffee. The governments of several countries are using technology to assist with helping warn people about exposure from people they were not aware by using GPS data or Wi-Fi location data. Even with technology to assist with notification of exposure, the wise and cautious must still maximize protective habits of hand hygiene and mask usage.

April 22, 2020

Autopsies in California now confirm something many have suspected for months … that people were infected with Coronavirus in January and February walking around and spreading the disease. Without widespread testing, it will be impossible in the future to identify everyone who is carrying the disease.

Everyone wants to know their COVID-19 status and learn if they have the virus now or had the virus in the past. How many tests will the country need to answer that question for 330 million people? One round of testing will most certainly be insufficient. Many factors complicate the calculations for how many tests will be needed. Most assuredly, many people will not be positive on the first test and they will need a second or third test when they develop illness in the future.

MYTH: If I'm exposed to COVID-19, I will develop antibodies to the virus that will protect me from future infection.

Antibodies develop during and after infection with COVID-19. Simply being exposed does not guarantee infection. Without infection, a person will likely not develop antibodies. Many people recall having a respiratory illness or other viral syndrome earlier this year, but only some of these were caused by COVID-19. Now that antibody testing is more available, we are starting to develop a clearer picture of the percentage of the population who have been infected with minimal or no symptoms.

Researchers released an analysis of the treatment of COVID-19 patients hospitalized in VA medical centers over the past 2 months. The study looked back and divided the patients into three groups, the patients who received hydroxychloroquine (HCQ) and azithromycin (AZ), the patients who received HCQ alone, and the ones who received neither. The hospital courses of over 350 patients were analyzed in this study. The death rate in the patients who received HCQ alone or HCQ and AZ was double the death rate in the patients who did not receive HCQ. This data is presented in a way to make you think that using HCQ can lead to higher death rate and lower chance of recovery. However, cause and effect relationships are not always so easy to establish.

When a person suffers a heart attack and goes to the hospital, the treatment given is determined by the severity of the heart attack. Patients with mild heart attacks are given medication while patients with severe heart attacks often undergo surgery or other invasive procedures. If you were to look back at a large group of both mild and severe heart attack patients, you might find that the death rate was higher in the group of patients with severe disease. You might even be led to believe that the surgery used to bypass blocked arteries is not effective because more people died in that group.

This is one of the shortcomings of looking backwards at complicated situations and trying to connect the dots – sometimes the wrong dots get connected. A group of patients with severe heart disease is more likely to die after treatment because the heart disease is severe, regardless of which method of treatment is given. Blaming the higher death rate on the type of treatment can only be done in a controlled prospective trial, a type of research study that looks forward and controls the situation so that there is only one major difference between the two groups being compared. Not all research studies are conducted equally, which means they do not all have the same level of validity. The studies with higher quality design will yield more relevant results, but you may have to rely on your doctor to help you see the differences.

April 23, 2020

We've known for weeks that the pandemic hit harder in New York than other parts of the country. We finally have some insight into how much more. A recent study reports about 20% a random sample of New Yorkers tested for COVID-19 antibodies were found to have them. This means that potentially up to 1 in 5 people in New York have been infected with COVID-19 and recovered.

People still have questions about what it means to be an asymptomatic carrier. Many diseases have a phase where a person has a disease and is unaware, because the disease has not yet caused any symptoms. Whether it's hypertension or HIV, our health system has adapted to check people regularly for diseases have little or no symptoms initially and are deadly if left untreated. We may see a similar approach with Coronavirus in the future if proper treatment or vaccination is not found this year.

April 24, 2020

Nearly 900,000 cases of infection and 50,000 lives lost after COVID-19 infection and all hopeful treatments are still in the testing stages. We are in the middle of a pandemic, but we are not so desperate that we should be poisoning ourselves attempting to cure a disease that most people do not yet have. Please do not ingest or inject into your body Lysol or any other cleaning agents. Just in case though, Poison Control can be reached by calling 1-800-222-1222 and is staffed 24 hours a day, 7 days a week.

MYTH: COVID-19 infection can be treated by drinking bleach or injecting yourself with bleach.

Bleach is appropriate for disinfection of surfaces, but it is poisonous to the human body if ingested or injected. No doctor or health expert of any kind will advise you to drink bleach or inject bleach for any reason, as this would poison your body. You should wear gloves to protect your skin when handling bleach and other harsh cleaning agents.

April 26, 2020

Concern is growing that the presence of antibodies may not mean immunity from disease. Logically, if a test for antibodies was invented last month for a disease we have never seen before, there can be no evidence on how long those antibodies last in the body and how well they will prevent future disease. Although this seems like common sense, there are some who are alarmed by this fact. It is possible that immunity last several months or several years, but it is unlikely that the antibodies will provide no immunity all.

Reportedly, a few countries are considering proposals for different versions of an "Immunity Pass" or "Immunity Passport" for individuals who have recovered after COVID-19 infection. Individuals who have recovered from COVID-19 may feel secure enough to travel, but governments are still likely to keep tight control over who enters across their borders regardless of their antibody status. Our country's government has banned people from over a dozen countries from entering the US and the list is likely to grow before it shrinks. Immunity passports are not likely to help people from the banned countries enter the US and likewise US citizens who have recovered from COVID-19 infection are probably not going to be allowed into countries with strict entry limitations such as New Zealand, Aruba, or Germany.

April 27, 2020

New York has released preliminary data on antibody test results from a random sample of residents that reveal upwards of 20% positive rate among New York City and a lower positive rate in upstate and rural areas of New York from 1-10%. These rates are higher than anticipated and suggest that their ability to test sick individuals may have been outpaced by the spread of the disease.

One person on a ship becomes infected with COVID-19. Soon after, several people are infected. Then, dozens of people, and sometimes hundreds of people become infected. The name of the ship has changed often, but the story is still the same. Is it even possible for any ship to be manned safely or is it time to abandon the idea of sea travel until vaccination or adequate outpatient treatment is available?

April 28, 2020

1 million cases of COVID-19 in the US and over 3 million cases worldwide. The virus seems unstoppable, but some countries have done well in slowing down the spread. My wife and I have always wanted to go to New Zealand. The landscapes look beautiful and visiting Hobbiton would be amazing. Unfortunately for us, that won't be happening anytime soon. New Zealand quickly implemented broad restrictions on any international arrivals to prevent anyone from bringing COVID-19 into their country.

Some people are trying to figure out how to resume school safely this fall. How will people react if a teacher coughs or a child runs a fever? How do you practice social distancing in a room full of Kindergarteners? If parents decide to keep their children home this fall until the situation has improved, will they continue while we wait collectively for a year or more while a vaccine is developed, tested, produced in mass quantities, and administered to the majority of the population? Will a country that doesn't fully embrace the flu vaccine be willing to accept a new vaccine with no previous safety record? Once the new vaccine is administered to early recipients, they must then be exposed to COVID-19 over a considerable amount of time to measure how effective the vaccine will be at preventing infection. The influenza vaccine prevents death from influenza much more than preventing influenza infection, and it is possible the COVID-19 vaccine might have the same effect.

While dozens of teams around the world work quickly to develop and test potential COVID-19 vaccines, it is still unlikely that a vaccine will be ready to distribute to the public. After safety trials and efficacy trials, a fast-track FDA approval by early 2021 is a realistic goal. Currently, most of the vaccines we use in the US for childhood vaccination are made in the US, Canada, France, Germany, Belgium, and Italy. Although the leaders of each country will desire their own population's protection, it would benefit everyone if several manufacturers worked together to implement mass production of the vaccine. Once vaccine manufacturing is announced, the race to obtain the product will begin.

Our leaders should start this year to develop a detailed distribution plan that will maximize prompt delivery of the vaccines in orderly fashion. Hopefully, our leaders have learned from facing the challenges of testing the public in mass numbers. Mass vaccination would require more locations than currently exist for mass testing, and it may require a higher level of training than what is needed for test administration. Public health departments will be strained if they attempt to vaccinate the entire population. The process should involve Pediatricians, Family Medicine physicians, Pharmacies, Urgent Care Clinics, and Hospitals so that the general public has a variety of options where they can receive vaccination. A logistics-based broad distribution plan could achieve vaccination of a majority of the US population within a year. European countries would be able to do the same, but in developing countries, the process could take twice as long or more.

April 30, 2020

People haven't been staying home just because of local government orders and national guidance from the White House and the CDC or out of concern for the greater good. Part of the reason people have been staying home and social distancing is fear of the disease and fear of death. As time passes, that fear wanes. As information and disinformation spreads, some people have less fear about exposing themselves to possible infection and more fear about what will happen if they continue to stay home to avoid that risk. If the risk of getting infected was a certain number, R, that risk will increase when people increase social contact. That increase in risk does not necessarily reduce simply be delaying the return to increased social interaction. Whether you wait 2 more days or 2 more weeks or 2 more months, COVID-19 will be waiting for us.

May 1, 2020

Nearly 3000 people died in the US today attributed to COVID-19. For months now, we have been watching daily counts increase. Our jaws hang collectively at death tolls that surpass losses during wars and yet we wonder about the accuracy of the data. In cities around the country, nursing homes and long-term care facilities are reporting historical increases in death, some of which are added to the total counts of COVID-19 related deaths as suspected or suspicious cases. Reporters and White House staff are being tested repeatedly, but we don't have enough tests for nurses. Whole prison units are being tested while city employees who keep our systems going are having difficulty getting tested. If we didn't have enough tests for the living, how could we possibly test all those who passed away?

MYTH: Health officials are purposely inflating the COVID-19 death toll with unrelated deaths to make the pandemic look worse than it really is.

Some people are casting doubt upon the COVID-19 tracking systems by claiming that many of the reported deaths are not really due to COVID-19. We already know that the virus can infect different organ systems and cause a vide range of symptoms in different people. Some patients develop respiratory failure, some develop blood clots in multiple blood vessels, and some develop other organ system failures. The limited quantity of COVID-19 disease tests forces every city and county to choose between testing to reduce future spread and testing to identify the current problem. Most cities have allocated tests in favor of testing sick individuals and given county medical examiners the flexibility to categorize deaths as COVID-related at their discretion. Each medical examiner typically has years of experience in their home county and can tell when a spike in deaths is unusual.

May 2, 2020

A report from the US Department of Homeland Security reveals intelligence information accusing China of misleading the world about the severity of the COVID-19 outbreak earlier this year. The reports details how China reduced exports of ventilators and medical supplies such as gloves and masks during January while importing those same items, theoretically to build up its inventory to fight against the COVID-19 outbreak. To shift from being an exporter of medical supplies to an importer in one month signals a coordinated effort likely led by the Chinese government to prepare for the worst while they downplayed the situation to the rest of the world.

The City of Houston is reporting that five Houstonians have died from COVID-19 in the past 24 hours, the highest number ever in Houston. Other cities with smaller populations have been reporting dozens or hundreds of deaths daily, which causes me to scrutinize this situation closely. Testing accuracy depends not only on the design of the test, but also its use. We know that tests for active disease become more accurate the longer the test subject has been sick. Influenza tests performed on people on Day 1 of illness often give false negative results, and some Chinese studies from mid-February of this year report a false negative rate of up to 30% in COVID-19 nasal swab PCR tests. The study highlighted the accuracy of any given test correlated somewhat with the severity of illness, meaning that tests were more likely to be accurate in patients with more severe illness and less likely to be accurate in patients with mild symptoms. The study also reported test accuracy was different depending on the type of sample on which the test was used. The accuracy of tests performed on sputum samples was higher than tests performed on nasopharyngeal swabs and the accuracy of tests performed on oropharyngeal (mouth) swabs was the lowest of them all.

We also know that test accuracy can be affected by operator error and inconsistencies in how a test is performed. When professional labs report test sensitivity and specificity, trained lab technicians are performing every step of each test with extreme caution to avoid any errors to maximize test accuracy. Learning how to administer a new test requires time and training. In the real world, newly trained clinic and hospital employees are likely more prone to making mistakes.

The recent stories from my patients and coworkers are disturbing. Patients who waited for hours for drive-up

COVID-19 nasal testing are reporting that they were handed the nasal swab and asked to swab themselves. Some of these patients were ill at the time but tested negative. The accuracy of nasal swab COVID-19 active disease tests depends on the quality of the nasal specimen collected. If the nasal swab comes out dry, the test could result in a false negative. Patients can also assist with the collection of a high-quality swab by remaining still during the collection process. It may feel uncomfortable, like a burning sensation, but the pain is worth it. A false-negative test doesn't help anyone.

Chapter 7

As the Death Toll Rises

You will notice quite often that media headlines will frequently contain the words "as the death toll rises" ... for example ... "City X loosens restrictions as the death toll rises" or "Major Official Y travels to Place Z as the death toll rises". I am not sure if this phrase is included to show things in a negative light, but it would be more honest to make clear to everyone that the death toll will always rise because death toll measures something that can only go up. This virus will continue to spread and unfortunate victims will lose their battle with this virus every day. Businesses and beaches will reopen as the death toll rises. Major sports leagues will return to competition as the death toll rises. Kids will return to daycare and school as the death toll rises. The world will go on as the death toll rises.

May 3, 2020

In a perfect world, every person infected with Coronavirus would notice their symptoms and get tested on the same day, and receive a perfectly accurate test that identifies all infected individuals every time, regardless of how early in the infection a person gets tested. In a perfect world, the people with positive tests will give the name and number of every person in close proximity to them over the previous week, including the people standing behind them unknowingly and even the people who happened to touch the same doorknob or elevator button, and each of those close contact would get the same perfect COVID-19 test for active disease. In a perfect world, each of these COVID-19 positive people will be able to self-isolate for the recommended 14 days without exposing family and friends to the disease and without the economic repercussions of missing two weeks of income. In a perfect world, every clinic and hospital would have adequate personal protective equipment to care for these patients and every ICU would have adequate supply of N95 respirators, ventilators, and other equipment to deliver the best anti-viral treatment to all patients to save as many lives as possible.

Our world is far from perfect. None of these things are happening perfectly, and these imperfections allow COVID-19 to continue to spread. Although the pandemic is far from over, there are some leaders declaring victory over Coronavirus in their area of jurisdiction. If you take the perspective that this fight against COVID-19 will be a marathon, celebrating successes at this point would be like doing a victory dance after mile 3 or 4. Great accomplishments have been made in the areas of improving testing and reducing the spread of infection, but the virus has not been stopped.

May 4, 2020

Several recent reports reveal the US Senate does not have adequate COVID-19 testing capability to test Senators and staff for infection as they reconvene for the Congressional session at the Capitol. This means that the US government does not have adequate testing equipment and supplies to effectively screen people to allow the US Senate to function. Workplaces around the country will facing a similar situation – navigating a reopening of business without adequate testing to screen out infected employees, contractors, and customers.

Meanwhile, in China, students are returning to school for traditional classroom instruction in several parts of the country. To reduce risk of spreading COVID-19, student's desks are spaced apart, children wear masks, and thermal scanners are used at the entrances to identify anyone with a fever. The world is watching to learn how best to provide quality education and keep them safe from infection.

MYTH: Taking temperature on arrival is a good way to screen for COVID-19.

Every place of business is looking for the best way to keep COVID-19 out and maintain a safe working environment. Most places are taking temperatures of everyone who arrives. The truth is that looking for fever or elevated temperature is not a good way to screen for COVID-19. It's true that some people with COVID-19 infection will develop a fever, but this is not always the case. Many people have fever without having COVID-19 and many people with COVID-19 will not develop a fever. Unfortunately, we don't have a cheaper way to identify sick individuals. Screening out people with fever is still a good idea because those people are probably sick with something.

May 8, 2020

Over 1000 Texans have died with COVID-19 infection since the epidemic began. Locally, the epidemic in Texas is still on the upswing. As stay at home orders are relaxed and business reopen that involve interacting with people closely, we should prepare for increases in infections. When social distancing and other prevention methods are effective, disease spreads slowly. When these measures are phased out, the disease will spread to more people at a steady pace, even in places where the disease has always been under control.

May 10, 2020

A research study conducted by the National Institute of Allergy and Infectious Disease that tested the effect of Remdesivir on hospitalized COVID-19 patients was halted prior to the expected end of the study. The good news is that Remdesivir works on critically ill. The bad news is that supply is limited worldwide and that the medicine can only be given intravenously at this time. The study included over

1000 patients admitted for hospital treatment of confirmed COVID-19 with respiratory illness symptoms. The patients were randomly assigned to the treatment group which received Remdesivir or the placebo group who did not. Both groups received similar standards of supportive care from the hospital. The preliminary results from the middle of the study revealed the Remdesivir group recovered from illness days faster and the death rate of patients in the Remdesivir group was lower. These benefits were significant enough for the study leaders to halt the study and give Remdesivir to both groups. Remdesivir is the first drug to show proven benefit for COVID-19 patients in a prospective randomized controlled trial and we hope that this is the first step toward the development of treatment that can be given to everyone.

May 11, 2020

Several White House staffers have tested positive for COVID-19 in the past week, which raises significant concerns about their infection prevention protocols. One of the President's personal valets at the White House has tested positive for COVID-19. Interestingly, this valet is not a vehicle driver who spends much of his time outside attending to cars. In the White House, valet is a title that has been used for people who perform many tasks, like a personal assistant or messenger. The details of the duties of this particular valet have not yet been disclosed, but this personal valet more likely traveled in and out of the White House frequently, and possibly worked near the President.

Coincidentally, the White House now requires staffers to wear masks at work. This announcement also shows that employees were not mandated to wear masks prior to this. Despite easy access to testing, and some people getting tested daily, we are seeing White House staffers test positive. Logically, one could make the deduction that widespread testing is not enough to prevent your workforce from getting COVID-19. If the White House cannot keep COVID-19 out of the workplace, what hope do everyday businesses have of achieving the same?

MYTH: Homemade masks offer no benefit to the wearer or the people around them.

It is true that all face coverings fulfill the basic function of containing the large droplets that are expelled when a person coughs or sneezes. For this reason, it is still advised for people to wear face coverings of any kind when you are in public but not able to distance yourself from others. Unfortunately, not every homemade mask will contain the smaller particles that can exit when breathing. Medical masks are made with multiple layers of filtration fibers to keep foreign particles out. Some homemade masks are made with similar filtration material but identifying them from the simple cloth masks can be tricky. A quick way to tell the difference is to see if you can blow through the mask to blow out a candle or a lighter. If the flame goes out, your mask does not have strong filtration, but if the flame does not move, your mask has adequate filtration.

Dr. Xavier Odili

May 15, 2020

California State University has announced that most classes this fall will be online. While there are some classes that can be taught adequately online, there are many that cannot. In the same way that a restaurant meal served on a hot plate with proper table service is not the same as eating it out of a to-go box, we know that in-person primary school education is not equivalent to an online variation of elementary school. We also know that online access and internet speed varies from person to person and differs based on the community in which you live, meaning that students will have unequal experiences with online education. All of these factors are being considered as our leaders determine the best way forward in the fall. The real question isn't just about returning to a normal school schedule in the fall, but whether or not parents are willing to do online learning for the next 2 years or so until an effective COVID-19 vaccine can be developed and distributed around the country.

MYTH: A vaccine will be ready for the general public by the end of 2020.

Everyone hopes that the process of developing a successful vaccine is much faster, but that would be the best-case situation, like winning the vaccine development lottery. But most people do not plan their lives around the hopes that they win the lottery. Most people plan for the future using actual information about the present. When vaccines are tested for safety, waiting a week and declaring them safe because no one died is not adequate. No one wants a vaccine that's only been tested for a week. Even when safety over several months has been established, there will not be any data on long term safety, and that will cause some people to pause, but researchers will proceed with testing the effectiveness of the vaccine.

During this phase, people will receive the vaccine and be monitored over time to see if they develop COVID-19. The rate of infection of the vaccinated people will be compared to the rate of infection in the general population to see how effective the vaccine is at preventing infection. These studies will also last several months because a vaccine that only prevents infection for a week or two is not a vaccine at all. After a few vaccines demonstrate initial effectiveness, the FDA will likely attempt to verify these results by reproducing the effect in a new group of volunteers to make sure that the best vaccine is put forward in hopes of protecting the country. These steps cannot be rushed, or rather, if they are rushed, the outcomes may not be the ones we are hoping for. Pretending that the process can be sped up is also not helpful to people trying to properly plan for the future.

Chapter 8

The Second Wave of COVID-19 Cometh

May 17, 2020

Every week the country will reach a new milestone in terms of cases of infection and numbers of lives lost. I can sense the fatigue people are feeling after daily coverage of this pandemic for 4 months straight. The fear of the unknown is fading, and people are venturing out more. Health officials will monitor for more subtle changes in the rate of how the death toll rises, looking for clues as to what types of activities are associated with greater spread of disease. In a similar fashion, each of us will have to evaluate the types of activities we continue in the future. Taking the family to a buffet restaurant will probably be a thing of the past. Lots of people will probably pass on going to the community pool as well. Shaking hands with strangers may never see a comeback. Movie theaters, cruise ships, and other crowded enclosed venues will continue to fall victim to COVID-19 until we develop better treatment or a vaccine.

Scientists are developing COVID-19 antigen tests in hopes of developing a more accurate way to identify people who are infected. Currently, we rely on viral tests using nasal or oral swabs to find infected people, but this only works when the disease has reached a certain phase when the virus can be detected by the tests. An antigen test looks for viral particles in the blood to verify infection. These viral particles can potentially be found much sooner than waiting for them to appear in the nose or mouth. There are already dozens of brands of tests already on the market, so adding a new class of testing isn't going to make things easier for patients to understand. However, if antigen testing becomes the faster and more reliable method of diagnosing COVID-19, everyone will benefit.

May 19, 2020

Early results from a vaccine trial show promise as vaccine recipients develop antibodies to COVID-19. The vaccine manufacturer Moderna has reported results on the first 8 individuals to receive their new vaccine currently under study. The truth is that 45 people participated in this trial, and the results of the other participants has not yet been released. The information that was released indicate that 8 individuals received two doses of vaccine and later developed antibodies to COVID-19. Typically, an experiment with only 8 participants would not yield significant results. In this case it is a beacon of hope. The first vaccine to be tested in humans appears safe over the short time period of monitoring.

While this is amazing news, the story isn't over. Verification is still an ongoing process and the effectiveness of antibodies has not yet been fully studied. When baking a turkey or a roast, you set the oven temperature and cook for an appropriate amount of time, but you still check the internal temperature during the process and check the food afterwards to ensure that it has properly cooked. If you served the food without double-checking, you would put the health of everyone eating at risk. The same is true for delivery of a vaccine. If the vaccine safety and effectiveness is not properly verified, everyone using the vaccine would be at risk.

May 22, 2020

Over 25,000 new cases of COVID-19 infection were reported in the past 24 hours. Over 5 million cases of infection worldwide and over 1.5 million in the US. With over 90,000 COVID-19 related deaths, more people have now died from COVID-19 in a few short months than any flu season of recent record. This is more than just a typical flu, and we are far from the end of this pandemic.

Malls may be dying away all over the country, but in Houston, malls are alive and well. I keep hearing from neighbors and patients that the malls have been packed ever since stay at home orders were lifted partially. It leads me to believe that our success with stay at home orders and controlling the spread of COVID-19 in Houston has fostered a false sense of security among Houstonians. The activities we once considered normal are no longer as safe as we would like. Riding in an Uber with strangers isn't very safe. Passing a hookah pipe around with your friends isn't that safe. Standing in a crowded elevator isn't that safe. Sharing sips of a drink with your girlfriends isn't that safe. Life as we know it isn't that safe anymore, and this is why you have to work that much harder to protect yourself from COVID-19.

May 25, 2020

On this Memorial Day, we honor those who gave their lives in defense of this country and we recognize that recently those warriors have not received proper burial honors due to the social limitations surrounding the COVID-19 pandemic. So many people have been unable to gather and lay their loved ones to rest in the past few months. So many people are suffering though this pandemic. Reports of domestic abuse are up. Donations of blood and blood products are down. Unemployment and bankruptcies are also going up. Although it seems like we are surrounded by sadness at times, there are things to be hopeful about. The waters of the canals in Venice are clearing up and sea life has returned there. Air pollution has dropped in different cities around the world allowing residents of Punjab, India to see the snow-capped peaks of the Himalayas and people in Nairobi, Kenya can see Mount Kenya again. American Astronauts returning to space from US soil for first time in years, hoping to leave COVID-19 behind.

US adds Brazil to list of travel ban countries as Brazilian cases of COVID-19 pass 325,000, more than any other country in the world except for the US. It's no surprise that a country with a densely packed urban population and a president who doesn't believe COVID-19 is a real threat is having a surge of infections. I don't know much about the healthcare system of Brazil, but I will still predict that pretending that the virus isn't serious is not going to help reduce the spread of disease.

May 26, 2020

The "Shutdown Syndrome" is in full effect now. Nearly every day, a patient comes in asking for COVID-19 testing because of a workplace exposure and a requirement to get tested before returning to work. Businesses and restaurants have an employee test positive, and they inform all employees and close down for a period of time. This all seems like reasonable actions, but what happens a week or two from now when another employee tests positive? We do not have enough tests to maintain multiple testing for a large number of employees on a rolling basis for the rest of the year. What business can stay open if it closes down for a week or two every month? What employee can survive if the office or restaurant where they work closes sporadically and decides not to pay employees while closed? What business can stay open while employees have tested positive and others may be asymptomatic carriers of infection? This situation has no easy answer, but we may not be able to sustain the current trend for long.

Almost every day, I see a patient who has been exposed to COVID-19 by a coworker who tested positive in the past few days. They all give a similar story, that the whole floor or the whole team has been sent home and told not to return until you have a negative COVID-19 test. This is the type of contact testing that must happen to prevent wild spread of the disease, but this also means that we will need more testing centers so that everyone has access to expedient testing that gives results in a reasonable amount of time.

June 1, 2020

A few short weeks ago, protesters lined the streets to voice their desire to be free from the economic shackles of Stay at Home orders. They had calculated the risks of going out amongst others without any face coverings, disregarding social distancing, and shouting in protest for hours. They were certain that the potential consequences of staying home and doing nothing was greater. It isn't hard to understand the desire to be free and to be able make life choices for yourself.

This week a different group of protesters are gathering in cities around the country for freedom as well. The images of a police officer sworn to protect and serve kneeling on the neck of a citizen in handcuffs while his own hands are in gloves cannot be ignored. This is a grave reminder of the fact that the fear of COVID-19 is not an excuse to forget about your humanity. People are again calculating the risks of going out and exposing themselves and comparing it to the risk of doing nothing. The desire for freedom from oppression and the freedom of living without fear of dying an unjust death is also easy to understand.

June 4, 2020

Thousands of people in dozens of cities around the country and around the world are shouting without masks in an exercise of freedom of speech. Social distancing seems like a forgotten practice. For over a week we have watched images of friends and neighbors protesting with strangers in solidarity, shoulder to shoulder against hate, and not a second thought about COVID-19. Life has a funny way of putting things in perspective. What seems like a big problem can suddenly seem small when an even bigger threat appears. The fear of dying from COVID-19 infection is being overshadowed by the fear of dying of hunger and fears of financial ruin, but now the fear of dying from an encounter with the police is also competing for that same portion of your attention. Some people say there are just a few bad apples. Others look at this situation and see an orchard of poisonous trees that have grown out of the bad apples of the past generations. Everyone should be able to agree that action is needed to stop the patterns of the past and move toward a brighter future.

June 5, 2020

New York City reports 0 confirmed deaths from COVID-19 for three days in a row now, which is something to celebrate. The curve was flattened successfully in New York by the persistence of their leaders and the adherence of New Yorkers to the guidelines recommended by the Governor. These results are proof that evidence-based recommendations and good leadership can conquer any dire situation.

Six months into the year 2020 and we are still closer to the beginning of this story than the end. It is important to draw distinction between exposure to COVID-19 and infection with COVID-19. More likely than not, if you are leaving your house, even on an occasional basis, you have been in close proximity with someone infected with COVID-19 without either of you knowing it. Make peace with this, and you will be able to focus on remaining vigilant. Exposure does not mean infection.

MYTH: If I am exposed to someone with COVID-19, I will most likely become infected with COVID-19.

Simply being in the presence of someone with COVID-19 does not guarantee infection. Through contact tracing and follow-up testing, we have seen that many people who were in close proximity to a confirmed COVID-19 patient never contract the viral illness. Many of the patients who come in for testing because of a coworker or friend they spent time with are testing negative and never develop symptoms. It's also important to seek a COVID-19 test at the appropriate time after exposure.

If you are around a large group of people without masks or you find out you were in close contact with someone who tested positive for COVID-19, fear may push you to get a test immediately. It would be more informative if you got that test a few days after your exposure. An early test may give a false negative test if the virus is present but has not replicated enough to be identified by the test.

Fortunately, rapid testing for active disease is more widely available. By testing and isolating quickly, we reduce the potential spread to others during the waiting period of uncertainty. You no longer have to wait a week in home isolation for your nasal swab test results. The ability to identify positive patients quickly will also lead to faster communication with the close contacts of the COVID-19 cases.

June 6, 2020

Studies that previously described risk of HCQ have been retracted. In medicine, we always strive to recommend treatment based on the best evidence, which comes from controlled studies that are monitored and then repeated to verify that results are consistent over time. The fear of being overwhelmed by the COVID-19 pandemic has created a situation where scientists are trying to cautiously rush forward to find new treatment options. Publishing a study and having it retracted is a byproduct of trying to speed through what is supposed to be a slow process.

June 10, 2020

As we approach 2 million confirmed cases of COVID-19, we can already measure significant increases in some parts of the country where stay at home orders were lifted a few weeks ago. Large social gatherings at beaches, bars, and clubs will likely result in the culmination of the second wave of COVID-19 infections. Hospitalizations of COVID-19 patient is also rising in many states, including Texas. In the Houston area, the trend of rising cases and rising hospitalizations is troubling. At the current rate of increase, the number of sick patients may exceed the hospital capacity to provide care, which is exactly the outcome our efforts were designed to prevent.

After everything we have lived through, there are still people who will say that COVID-19 is a hoax. Similarly, there are people who believe the earth is flat. If you want to see what happens to a community with no social distancing, no stay at home regulations, and minimal mask usage, research the news reporting how the COVID-19 pandemic is affecting our Native American communities. A friend of mine left the hustle and bustle of Houston back in January for a simpler life as a nurse on a Native American Reservation in Arizona. She gives us updates from time to time and her stories match up with the ones reported on the news. Life there has not been so simple. The virus is running rampant and the people are not heeding the warnings from the CDC and other government agencies. The mistrust of government that began generations ago has not died down even though the infection rates are some of the highest in the country.

This is not the time for complacency. We all understand the need to interact with each other for the benefit of our families, our businesses, and our own personal benefit. You don't need to wait for this virus to harm your friends or family to start to take this seriously. You can fight against the spread of the disease right now. Our actions must be taken safely for the benefit of everyone. Just like the first wave rose and fall, we will adapt and the second wave will recede, but only if we act with appropriate caution and protective behavior. When this storm has passed, and we reach a calm state again, we must encourage everyone to be cautious and responsible in the fall, or we may find that the third wave is even worse than the first two.

APPENDIX

The Myth and Facts of Coronavirus

Myth: The Coronavirus can only live for a few hours on common surfaces.

FACT: A scientific study conducted by the CDC, NIH, UCLA, and Princeton University published in the New England Journal of Medicine in March tells a different story. Researchers demonstrated that the virus was found on copper surfaces 4 hours later, on cardboard 24 hours later, and on plastic and stainless-steel surfaces up to 72 hours later.

Myth: The Coronavirus is an airborne illness that can live in the air for days.

FACT: The virus spreads through small particles carried by respiratory droplets when an infected person sneezes or coughs but that spread occurs within 6-9 feet of that person. If you share a room with a person but remain a good distance away, you are not at any significant risk of getting the virus.

Myth: "Flattening the curve" means that we reduce the number of cases of infection and we return to normal life faster.

FACT: To flatten the curve means to slow down the pace of infections, spread the infections out over a longer time-period so that hospitals are not overwhelmed.

Myth: I should wear an N95 respirator or surgical facemask and protect myself from Coronavirus infection.

FACT: There is no evidence that individual members of the public will reduce their risk of infection by wearing a high-level respirator. In fact, most people have not been shown how to properly use or wear a respirator or surgical facemask. Instead, they may provide a false sense of reassurance and also cause people to touch their face more than if they were not wearing a mask. The CDC is now recommending that people wear face coverings and handmade masks to help keep people from spreading viral particles if they happen to be infected and not know it. Wearing a face covering of any kind will limit the spread of viral particles from infected people and that will help protect everyone. It is possible that universal mask usage may be recommended if the country were to have adequate supply and adequate education on correct use. Proper hand washing and avoidance of face contact with unclean hands are the best ways to prevent infection.

Myth: Drinking sips of hot tea or hot water will wash Coronavirus down into your stomach and prevent you from getting the illness.

FACT: While staying well hydrated is good for your general health, there is no evidence that hydrating with hot liquids every 15 minutes will reduce risk of infection with Coronavirus or any other infectious disease.

MYTH: Warm weather will kill the virus and stop the outbreak of Coronavirus.

FACT: We do not know how warmer temperatures will affect the spread of COVID-19. It would be nice if it just disappeared after winter ends, but I would not bet on it.

Myth: Coronavirus is transmitted by drinking Corona beer.

FACT: There is no Coronavirus in Corona beer or any other beverage.

Myth: No one predicted another worldwide pandemic. No one could have seen this coming.

FACT: Intellectuals have been ringing alarm bells for years about how the world is not prepared for the next pandemic infection. No one talks about earthquakes as if there will never be another earthquake. No one talks about war as if there will never be another war. We watch and prepare and practice with drills for

earthquakes and wars and now even active shooters. Experts will tell you that we should have been preparing for the next pandemic as well.

Myth: Cats and dogs can become infected with Coronavirus and spread the infection to humans.

FACT: Scientists and researchers do not have sufficient evidence to establish spread between humans and pets or any other animals. There are isolated reports of a single animal testing positive without exhibiting symptoms, which may simply be asymptomatic carrier state without any proof of spread of disease.

Myth: Africans and African Americans are immune to Coronavirus.

FACT: Although we did not receive reports of large outbreaks in Africa in the Spring that were similar to the ones in Asia, Europe, and the US, there are thousands of people of African descent with COVID-19.

Myth: Children and young people are immune to the effects of Coronavirus.

FACT: Although the majority of severe cases of Coronavirus infection occur in the elderly, there are several reports of children needing ICU care after Coronavirus infection. Studies evaluating COVID-19 hospitalized patients in the US show 20% of hospitalized cases involve patients between the ages of 20 and 44. Children and young people can be severely affected by this virus.

Myth: As long as I wear gloves whenever I'm out, I won't get Coronavirus.

FACT: Gloves are good for protecting your hands from touching viruses and bacteria on surfaces. However, if you grab your cell phone while wearing gloves, you have just spread those germs to your phone. If you touch your face while wearing those gloves, you have just defeated the purpose of wearing the gloves. It's important to remember that no one thing will protect you fully and that you must combine good habits to have the best protection possible.

Myth: I can protect myself from Coronavirus by gargling with bleach and water.

FACT: There is no benefit to rinsing or gargling or drinking bleach in any form. Please do not expose yourself to danger by drinking bleach or any other dangerous chemicals.

Myth: Lysol spray will kill Coronavirus in midair.

FACT: It's understandable that everyone wants to do everything they can to protect themselves, but I have to say that I am tired of walking into a room and

breathing in from a cloud of Lysol Disinfectant Spray. The instructions on the can clearly state exactly which types of surfaces can be cleansed with the spray. That's right ... surfaces. Hard surfaces, soft surfaces, semi-porous surfaces ... but nothing about killing anything in the air. After spraying onto your surface of choice, it is equally important to let the spray stand for the necessary amount of time to properly kill the germs. Wiping the Lysol away does not kill the germs. The amount of time you need to wait depends on the germs you are intending to kill. Most germs are killed in 2 minutes, but some require ten minutes. This means you need to spray and walk away if you want to use Lysol correctly.

Myth: I should avoid Ibuprofen and other anti-inflammatory medications because taking them can make my infection with Coronavirus even worse.

FACT: There is no evidence that any over the counter medication like Advil, Motrin, Ibuprofen, Tylenol, or Acetaminophen cause worse outcomes in patients with Coronavirus. Although the Health Minister of France advised the French people to avoid using anti-inflammatory medicines such as Advil or Motrin the risks of complications are not certain. Severe cases of Coronavirus infection could indirectly lead to kidney damage and high dose use of non-steroid anti-inflammatory medicines could also cause kidney damage. In most cases, patients who are critically ill are not taking over-the-counter medication at the same time. If you have kidney damage, you should be avoiding these medicines already. Most people with Coronavirus infection will not develop kidney failure and do not need to avoid Ibuprofen and other similar medicines.

Myth: I can use a blow dryer to blow hot air into my nostrils to kill germs and protect me from Coronavirus.

FACT: There is no evidence that applying hot air to the nostrils or breathing in steam provides any protection from Coronavirus or any other infection.

Myth: 4 out of every 5 people are already carriers for Coronavirus.

FACT: Looking back at the first wave, COVID-19 had only affected a small percentage of Americans, less than 10% actually. Although we cannot see everyone who has the virus, we are certain that the prevalence of the disease was nowhere near 80%.

Myth: My town doesn't have any cases of Coronavirus, so I don't have to worry about getting the virus when I'm out in public.

FACT: Although your town may not have any reported cases of COVID-19 now, that may change at any time. If your county does not test aggressively, they may not

pick up on the infection that is already there. People travel from the city to small towns all the time and may bring the virus with them. And if your county does not have a major hospital, people who are sick and live in your county will probably drive to a bigger county, get tested, and be reported there. It's safer for now for you to protect yourself until the pandemic is under control.

Myth: Because I don't have cough or fever, I probably don't have Coronavirus.

FACT: There is no strict set of symptoms that determine if someone has a Coronavirus infection. Some people have fever and cough, while others do not. Some people have chills and body aches. Some even report vomiting and diarrhea. It is even possible to have the virus and have no symptoms of illness for several days.

Myth: The better we adhere to social distancing, the faster we will eradicate Coronavirus.

FACT: Some patients still believe that after 2 or 4 or 6 weeks of social distancing, the virus will disappear, and life will return to normal. Unfortunately, the opposite is true. The virus will continue to spread until there are enough people with immunity to interrupt the chain of transmission. Social distancing slows down the spread of infection thereby slowing the development of natural immunity. Effective social distancing practices extend the life of the epidemic over a longer time period. Under these guidelines, people will not be able to develop natural immunity rapidly unless a vaccine is developed rapidly. Worldwide there more than 750,000 cases of Coronavirus infection and over 150,000 cases in the United States. There are so many people infected, that it will be nearly impossible for the virus to be eradicated this year. There will always be parts of society that must continue to interact closely with others, and thus, the virus will seek to hang on to that foothold.

Myth: If I test negative for Coronavirus, I'm clear from disease and I don't have to worry about being infected.

FACT: Patients who test negative at one point in time may be exposed to the virus in the future and contract the disease. It is also possible to test negative for disease but have the virus in your system at an early stage of infection. A negative test provides information about the past, not necessarily about the present, and surely not about the future. No test is perfect. All testing is flawed in some way. A clinician must learn the flaws of a test in order to use the test properly. You should always discuss your test results with your provider to better understand the full meaning of those results.

Myth: All COVID-19 antibody tests are faulty and prone to give false positive or false negative results.

FACT: No test is perfect. It's reasonable to have concern about the accuracy of any test that you take. A pregnancy test will always be validated by an ultrasound later. A screening HIV test will be validated by a second confirmatory test. A mammogram that suggests a tumor will be validated by a biopsy. We already understand that every test has a risk of false results. The real question should be how much is that risk of false results. Only the data can answer that question. Fears are rising among the public after reports of several COVID-19 tests being sold with high rates of test result inaccuracies. I have read about the fears, but I have not seen any data showing high rates of false results. Data is data. However, if someone is concerned, that person can request and read the data behind a test, or at least ask someone who has read the data. Antibody testing is not an emergency need. If someone is afraid, they should not take a test they do not trust. As research continues, testing accuracy will improve, and better tests will hopefully be developed here in the USA.

Myth: If I'm exposed to COVID-19, I will develop antibodies to the virus that will protect me from future infection.

FACT: Antibodies develop during and after infection with COVID-19. Simply being exposed does not guarantee infection. Without infection, a person will likely not develop antibodies. Many people recall having a respiratory illness or other viral syndrome earlier this year, but only some of these were caused by COVID-19.

Now that antibody testing is more available, we are starting to develop a clearer picture of the percentage of the population who have been infected with minimal or no symptoms.

Myth: COVID-19 infection can be treated by drinking bleach or injecting yourself with bleach.

FACT: Bleach is appropriate for disinfection of surfaces, but it is poisonous to the human body if ingested or injected. No doctor or health expert of any kind will advise you to drink bleach or inject bleach for any reason, as this would poison your body. You should wear gloves to protect your skin when handling bleach and other harsh cleaning agents.

Myth: Health officials are purposely inflating the COVID-19 death toll with unrelated deaths to make the pandemic look worse than it really is.

FACT: Some people are casting doubt upon the COVID-19 tracking systems by claiming that many of the reported deaths are not really due to COVID-19. We already know that the virus can infect different organ systems and cause a vide range of symptoms in different people. Some patients develop respiratory failure, some develop blood clots in multiple blood vessels, and some develop other organ system failures. The limited quantity of COVID-19 disease tests forces every city and county to choose between testing to reduce future spread and testing to identify the current problem. Most cities have allocated tests in favor of testing sick individuals and given county medical examiners the flexibility to categorize deaths as COVID-related at their discretion. Each medical examiner typically has years of experience in their home county and can tell when a spike in deaths is unusual.

Myth: Taking temperature on arrival is a good way to screen for COVID-19.

FACT: Every place of business is looking for the best way to keep COVID-19 out and maintain a safe working environment. Most places are taking temperatures of everyone who arrives. The truth is that looking for fever or elevated temperature is not a good way to screen for COVID-19. It's true that some people with COVID-19 infection will develop a fever, but this is not always the case. Many people have fever without having COVID-19 and many people with COVID-19 will not develop a fever. Unfortunately, we don't have a cheaper way to identify sick individuals. Screening out people with fever is still a good idea because those people are probably sick with something.

Myth: Homemade masks offer no benefit to the wearer or the people around them.

FACT: It is true that all face coverings fulfill the basic function of containing the large droplets that are expelled when a person coughs or sneezes. For this reason, it is still advised for people to wear face coverings of any kind when you are in public but not able to distance yourself from others. Unfortunately, not every homemade mask will contain the smaller particles that can exit when breathing. Medical masks are made with multiple layers of filtration fibers to keep foreign particles out. Some homemade masks are made with similar filtration material but identifying them from the simple cloth masks can be tricky. A quick way to tell the difference is to see if you can blow through the mask to blow out a candle or a lighter. If the flame goes out, your mask does not have strong filtration, but if the flame does not move, your mask has adequate filtration.

Myth: A vaccine will be ready for the general public by the end of 2020.

FACT: Everyone hopes that the process of developing a successful vaccine is much faster, but that would be the best-case situation, like winning the vaccine development lottery. But most people do not plan their lives around the hopes that they win the lottery. Most people plan for the future using information about the present. When vaccines are tested for safety, waiting a week and declaring them safe because no one died is not adequate. No one wants a vaccine that's only been tested for a week. Even when safety over several months has been established, there will not be any data on long term safety, and that will cause some people to pause, but researchers will proceed with testing the effectiveness of the vaccine.

Myth: If I am exposed to someone with COVID-19, I will most likely become infected with COVID-19.

FACT: Simply being in the presence of someone with COVID-19 does not guarantee infection. Through contact tracing and follow-up testing, we have seen that many people who were in close proximity to a confirmed COVID-19 patient never contract the viral illness. Many of the patients who come in for testing because of a coworker or friend they spent time with are testing negative and never develop symptoms. It's also important to seek a COVID-19 test at the appropriate time after exposure.

Myth: Face masks interfere with your oxygen level.

FACT: Surgeons and surgical staff have been wearing masks 10 hours a day or more for decades with no reports of staff losing consciousness due to low oxygen level. The size of an oxygen molecule is approximately 0.1 nanometer (1×10^{-9} meter) in diameter. The pore size of an N95 respirator is 0.1 to 0.3 microns (1×10^{-6} meter) wide. The pores of standard surgical masks and cloth fabric masks are even larger. This means that oxygen molecules are 1000 times smaller than the spaces between fabric of any mask and oxygen can flow freely past any mask you wear.

Myth: The second wave of COVID-19 infections is a result of cities reopening too quickly.

FACT: The rise in number of COVID-19 infections is linked to the type and manner of social interactions, not dependent on the timeframe. Whether a city waits 2 more weeks or 2 more months, if the people in the city begin to mingle and interact without masks or social distancing, the number of infections will rise. Without an effective vaccine to prevent infections, a second wave was always going to happen, and more waves will come after that.

Thank you for reading!

Visit http://thebp.site/228081 or www.apexurgentclinic.com/about-us/ for info on digital downloads and how to order additional copies from the publisher, The Book Patch, or from amazon.com.

www.ingramcontent.com/pod-product-compliance
Lightning Source LLC
Chambersburg PA
CBHW070641220526
45466CB00001B/248